DRIVE

DRIVE

NEUROBIOLOGICAL AND MOLECULAR MECHANISMS OF SEXUAL MOTIVATION

DONALD W. PFAFF

A BRADFORD BOOK

THE MIT PRESS

CAMBRIDGE, MASSACHUSETTS

LONDON, ENGLAND

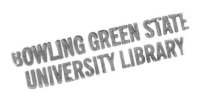

This book was set in Bembo by Northeastern Graphic Services, Inc., and was printed and bound in the United States of America.

Library of Congress Cataloging-in-Publication Data

Pfaff, Donald W., 1939–
     Drive : neurobiological and molecular mechanisms of sexual
motivation / Donald W. Pfaff.
        p. cm. — (Cellular and molecular neuroscience)
     "A Bradford book."
     Includes bibliographical references and index.
     ISBN 0-262-16184-2 (hc : alk. paper). — ISBN 0-262-66147-0
(pb : alk. paper). — ISBN 0-262-16184-2 (hc.)
     1. Sex (Biology)   2. Sexual excitement.   3. Neuropsychology.
4. Neuroendocrinology.   I. Title.   II. Series: Cellular and
molecular neuroscience series.
     [DNLM: 1. Sex Hormones—physiology.   2. Sex Behavior—physiology.
3. Sex Behavior, Animal—physiology.   4. Sex Hormones—genetics.
5. Neurobiology.   WK 900 P523d 1999]
QP251.P467   1999
573.6—dc21
DNLM/DLC
for Library of Congress   98-43055
                                                              CIP

CONTENTS

Contents

Contents

In the middle of this century, some of the neuroanatomical and electrophysiological tools necessary to launch a serious study of the central nervous system were just becoming available, but what we actually knew could be characterized as a tiny island in a vast sea of ignorance. Things have changed. Since that time, the cell-to-cell connectivities and the electrical properties of nerve cells, glial cells, and almost all their parts have been studied eagerly and exhaustively. In addition, discoveries about chemical neurotransmitters and neuropeptides in the brain have allowed us to use modern tools of biochemistry to acquire more insights into how the central nervous system works. Even more exciting, the DNA revolution has made relatively simple the application of the concepts and techniques of today's molecular biology to elucidating how the brain governs behavior.

In our own laboratory, we have been able to pinpoint some targets for hormone action in the brain. Most important, by revealing the first basic working neural circuit for a vertebrate behavior, we showed that such a task could be accomplished. But to what extent can the explanations of brain mechanisms and behavior in animals be used to explain some elements of human behavior? Here we claim that the biological bases for the most primitive human instincts are explained largely by mechanisms uncovered in animal brains that have not changed appreciably in their most fundamental properties over millions of years of evolution. This situation allows discovery of the neural and endocrine basis of the most primitive aspect of human sex drive, libido.

For two reasons, I have tried to keep this book simple. First, if the data and arguments are truly conclusive, then they should submit to a transparent, clear book-length presentation. Second, as a scientist supported by public funds, I believe I have the obligation to elucidate this area of neurobiological work well enough that students and educated laypeople can understand it. Therefore, far from writing for my colleagues, I am depending on them (see later) to help me to get the main points right so that the major message of brain and hormone mechanisms governing behavior will be easily understandable.

A pressing need arose during the last decade to summarize in the clearest way the tremendous progress in our field of neurobiology. Molecular genetic techniques have been incorporated into our field without loss of focus on important physiological and behavioral questions. Thus, we can begin with broad questions about certain aspects of behavior, dive into a rather detailed summary of neurobiological and molecular analyses, and emerge with answers that appear general enough to apply to a range of animals and humans.

We will not need to review large sets of facts on neural circuits; these were published previously in *Estrogens and Brain Function* (Pfaff, 1980) and supplemented in *The Physiology of Reproduction* (Knobil & Neill, 1994). Instead, we can explore new results on how genetic and physiological mechanisms are orchestrated in a virtual symphony to ensure that reproductive behaviors begin under optimum conditions. As examples of genetic effects, sex differences in brain and behavior will play a significant role in the book.

In the recent past, attention has been paid, on the one hand, to behavior for its own sake and, on the other hand, to molecular genetic forays. Our new book will show a surprising degree of accomplishment at the intersection where molecular genetics can serve neurobiology and behavior.

ACKNOWLEDGMENTS

This book represents a confluence of several creative forces. My teachers at Harvard University and the Massachusetts Institute of Technology (MIT) filled my days with useful instruction about brain function and the experimental analysis of behavior. In particular, Professors Joseph Altman and Walle J.H. Nauta were inspiring in their histochemical forays into neural circuits. Not incidentally, my first exposure to the concepts of psychoanalysis, one of which is explained here, occurred during those years. Cross-registration into Harvard Medical School, from graduate school at MIT, allowed exposure to some of the greatest minds and experimentalists in neurophysiology, including Professors Steven Kuffler, Torsten Wiesel, and David Hubel. Instruction there in the chemistry and physiology of the endocrine organs and their hormones served as part of my introduction to the steroid sex hormones, whose simple chemistry permitted us entrée to certain brain mechanisms and whose protein receptors brought us, without much additional effort, into modern eukaryotic molecular biology. At Rockefeller University, Professor Neal Miller served as a model of clear thinking about neural mechanisms for behavior, while Professors George Palade, Joshua Lederberg, Gerald Edelman, and Stanford Moore provided continuing inspiration. Most of all, the laboratory at Rockefeller University has been blessed with a large number of brilliant and talented individuals whose accomplishments comprise the experimental results and thoughtful interpretations included in the arguments presented here.

Throughout, I have relied on many friends and colleagues for good advice. I am indebted to the following for their willingness to read and criticize parts or all of the book. For expertise in molecular endocrinology, I have appreciated the reactions of Richard Lyttle, vice president for discovery at Wyeth-Ayerst, Dr. Barbara Attardi of Cornell Medical School, and Professor George Stancel of the department of pharmacology at the University of Texas Medical Center at Houston. For criticisms of the neurophysiology, I am grateful to Professor Victor J. Wilson at Rockefeller University and to Professor Yasuo Sakuma of Nippon University Medical School in Tokyo. For advice regarding the neuroanatomy, I thank Professor Naomi Rance in the department of pathology at the University of Arizona School of Medicine, Dr. Joan King, professor and chair of the department of anatomy at Tufts Medical School, and Dr. Miles Herkenham, chief of the section on functional neuroanatomy at the National Institute of Mental Health. Dr. John Russell, head of the department of physiology at the University of Edinburgh, was invaluable as a source of new material and criticisms about oxytocin gene expression, especially in relation to stress. For useful comments regarding trophic actions of hormones on neurons, I thank Professor Kathryn J. Jones of the University of Illinois School of Medicine. Professor James Matthews, in the department of psychology at New York University, has advised me about motivational theory, while Professor Randall R. Sakai of the University of Pennsylvania has been keen on the subject of hormone-stimulated mechanisms in the brain. Dr. Uriel Halbreich of the biobehavioral program in the department of psychiatry at State University of New York Medical School (Buffalo), and Dr. David Rubinow, chief of the behavioral endocrinology branch at the National Institute of Mental Health, have given good reactions regarding our extrapolations from animal to human brain and behavior. Dr. Ruth Guyer, science writer in Bethesda, Maryland, was helpful in her remarks about writing a book for a general audience. For excellent editorial advice on style and exposition, I thank Lucy Frank at the Rockefeller University.

I

INTRODUCTION

Questions addressed by the book, from molecular biology to behavior. Also showing how molecular and neurobiological findings play into questions of human drive.

Features of Drive, or Motivation:

"A central neural state of an organism" (Morgan, 1943)

"Both general and particular" (Bolles, 1967)

"Fundamentally, drives energize behavior" (Hull, 1943)

"Drives can direct activity toward goals" (Young, 1936)

1

QUESTIONS AND ARGUMENTS

You must remember this. A kiss is but a kiss. A sigh is but a sigh.
The fundamentals still apply. As time goes by.

—"As Time Goes By," in *Casablanca*, 1942

For centuries, people have been wondering about themselves, about their true nature. What makes them the way they are? Why do they do the things they do? What *animates* behavior? Indeed, this is the most fundamental question about behavior and its control by the brain: Why do we do anything at all? Concepts and experiments addressing brain mechanisms of motivation, or *drive,* should answer this question.

Even as tremendous attention has been centered on how animals and humans change their behavior by learning and memory, we must understand first the most elementary form of "neural plasticity," the very awakening of behavioral responses from a previously inactive person. *Drive* is a name for neural states that energize and direct behavior.

Clearly, a single book or a single set of research programs will not answer global questions about human personality. However, where should the neurobiologist start? The research summarized here addresses elementary questions

about a well-chosen, simple animal model. The answers explain a complete social behavior, which heuristically can be considered as an exemplar for motivated
behaviors: That is, the principles and findings discovered with sex hormone–
driven behaviors can be compared to other drives in lower animals and to the
most primitive sexual urges of humans. Experimental comparisons of this sort
should generate questions of interest to neurobiologists in the twenty-first
century.

The purpose of this chapter is to identify the questions and topics addressed throughout the book. Applying the fundamental question of the activation of behavior to the issue of sex drive, the neural circuitry (chapter 6) and
genes (chapter 7) have been analyzed well enough to explain how sex behavior responses are evokable from previously inactive animals. Here and throughout the book, the use of the word *animals* is meant to denote "infrahuman"
animals as distinct from human beings.

The entire book emphasizes the primacy of primitive urges to press the
point that, as far as humans are concerned, feelings and desires are important.
Even in the recent past, humans were often considered to be absolutely
unique in light of their information-processing abilities. Now, computers have
passed us by in all measures of mnemonic and calculating capacities. As any
"Star Trek" devoteé ("Trekkie") knows, we are more exquisitely human by
virtue of our desires and emotions. So, let us try to understand those human
features.

Figures 1.1 and 1.2 provide a brief, simplified introduction to some of
the mechanisms presented in later chapters. These mechanisms facilitate or restrain sex drive, respectively. Introduced in this chapter is the material covered
in the later chapters, question by question and point by point.

A. NEUROANATOMY OF DRIVE

How can we comprehend, in biological terms, why animals and human beings
initiate behaviors at some times and not others? To accomplish this, we need
to encounter the neural mechanisms of motivation, or drive. Here, we present

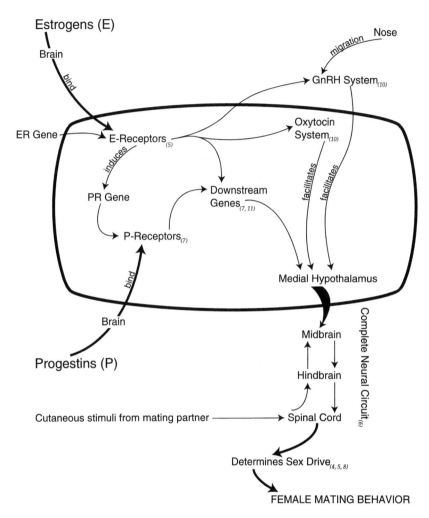

Figure 1.1 A simplified introduction to some of the hormonal, molecular, and neuronal "forces" that *facilitate* female-typical sex drive and mating behavior. Chapter numbers covering this material are shown in italics, in small brackets. Some of the influences that *limit* mating behavior are introduced in figure 1.2. As only a few of the topics covered are represented in this figure, some readers might also skip forward to chapter 9 (see figure 9.1).

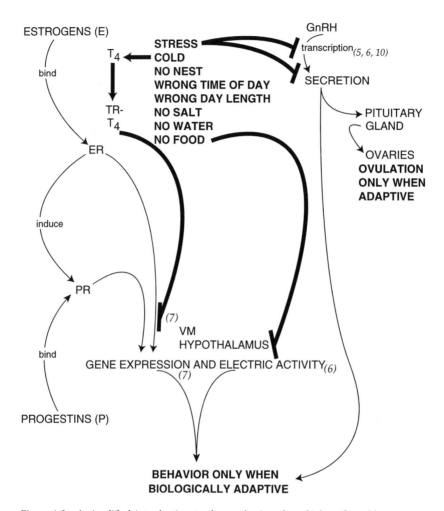

Figure 1.2   A simplified introduction to the mechanisms by which unfavorable environmental and physiological conditions can *restrain* mating behavior by limiting the operations of the mechanisms introduced in figure 1.1. Chapter numbers covering this material are shown in italics, in small brackets. A more complete summary is represented in figure 9.2.

a two-component theory of drive (see chapter 4). Its general component—
arousal—energizes behavior and depends on noradrenergic and dopaminergic
pathways, elucidated brilliantly by Swedish neuroanatomists some years ago.
These two types of nerve cell pathways (noradrenergic and dopaminergic) use
specific neurotransmitters—noradrenalin and dopamine—secreted from their
terminals to affect the next nerve cells in the pathways. Tomas Hökfelt, Kjell
Fuxe, Annika Dahlstrom, and their collaborators at the Karolinska Institutet in
Stockholm discovered in the brainstem systems of neurons that use these transmitters and that can "light up" the forebrain. The other component of drive is
particular for different biological needs. In this component of motivation, sex
drive uses different mechanisms to guide behavior than, for example, does
hunger drive. Because of great successes recently in molecular endocrinology,
the greatest progress in understanding motivation systems has been in the area
of explaining sex drive in animals and humans (see chapter 5).

1. Hormone Binding by Hormone Receptors

We have discovered systems of hormone-sensitive neurons that appear to be
present in the brains of all vertebrates, from fish to philosophers (see chapter 5).
These hormone-sensitive neurons contain specialized proteins, termed *hormone
receptors,* that have the property of strongly binding specific hormones. Initially,
these neurons were revealed by studies with radioactive hormones. Follow-up
studies with immunocytochemistry (a technique that uses brain tissue sections
to identify proteins in individual neurons) and molecular techniques [to measure gene products (messenger RNAs), which travel from the cell nucleus to the
cytoplasm to direct protein synthesis] have confirmed our conclusions. These
systems of hormone-binding neurons are found within the hypothalamus (a
small, primitive brain region that governs many hormonal systems, visceral reactions, and behavior) and the most ancient part of the forebrain, a region called
the *limbic system.*

In the hypothalamus and limbic system, sex hormones have at least two
kinds of effects on these hormone-receiving neurons. First, hormones change

gene expression in these cells and, in doing so, they alter which portion of our DNA—our genetic inheritance—is allowed to determine the panoply of proteins that actually operate the neuron. The importance of these changes is confirmed by hormone receptor gene "knockouts" through which important bits of DNA simply are deleted or disabled (chapter 7). Second, sex hormones have rapid electrical effects on cell membranes (see chapter 5). But, for meaningful behavioral effects, sex hormones cannot simply "be there." Such factors as how suddenly they appear, the order of their appearance, and the patterns of their breakdowns all help to determine what the behavioral consequences will be (see chapter 5).

Always, hormonal signals interact with external stimuli to control behavior (see chapter 6). In fact, we can see how these interactions satisfy the obvious (i.e., axiomatic) biological requirements for the drive toward reproduction and the limits on reproduction. In lower animals, hormones account for a larger slice of the causal pie, as compared to the greater importance of cultural influences in humans. The concerted effects of hormones and external stimuli on the brain beautifully synchronize reproductive controls in the pituitary (the master gland that hangs off the bottom of the hypothalamus) with reproductive behavior (chapter 6).

In sum, we establish the principle that hormones can powerfully determine behavior through specific chemical steps, depending on hormone receptors in specific parts of the brain.

2. NEURAL EXPLANATION

How are hormone effects in limbic and hypothalamic neurons (introduced earlier) transformed into a behavioral effect? A hormone-sensitive neural circuit has been discovered (Pfaff et al., 1994; see chapter 6). It is composed of separate modules: The *spinal cord module* handles "local business," the immediate sensorimotor reflexes involved; the *hindbrain module* coordinates activities across spinal levels; the *hypothalamic module* adds the hormone dependence; and the *midbrain module* provides the transition from sluggish neuroendocrine mechanisms of the hypothalamus to the motor control hierarchy of the hindbrain (see figures 1.1 and 6.1). This first neural circuit for an actual mammalian behavior establishes how behavior can be controlled by a series of specific neural mechanisms (see chapter 6).

3. Behavior Is Determinable

With a simple enough behavior of clear biological importance, it is possible to see that behavior is determined by biophysical and molecular mechanisms (see chapters 6 and 7). As introduced already, mechanisms laid bare by modern analytical techniques mediate the action of hormones, together with environmental stimuli, as they create on impact on the central nervous system. When these neural and molecular mechanisms are brought into play, reproductive behavior is initiated (see figure 1.1). Extrapolating from animal brains to human brains, we argue in chapter 8 that the application of systematic neurobiological thinking and methodology to human behaviors will reveal, in the twenty-first century, our scientific opportunities for explaining the simplest human urges. Where can our own feelings and actions be reduced to strict biological terms and wherein lies our unique psychological individuality?

4. A Series of Responses Feeding Forward

Within and around the relevant neural circuit, a symphony of neural adaptations assures smooth behavioral performance. Even before actual sex behaviors begin, a series of hormone-dependent communications between male and female constitute a sort of "behavioral funnel" ensuring that reproductively competent conspecifics—and only they—get together. In fact, the preliminary social behaviors leading to reproduction use an elegant neurophysiological mechanism. Two groups of nerve cells in the lower brainstem, the lateral vestibular nucleus and the medullary ventral reticular formation, exert tremendously powerful controls over our large postural muscles. They communicate with the spinal cord via, respectively, the lateral vestibulospinal and reticulospinal tracts. It turns out that courtship behaviors exhibited by the estrogen and progesterone-primed female massively activate the very vestibulospinal and reticulospinal tracts that then will be required for female mating behavior (see chapter 6).

B. Genes in the Nervous System Controlling Behavior

The tools of modern molecular biology have just begun to let us see how both hormonal controls on genes and (conversely) the effects of genetic background on hormonal actions can influence hormone-sensitive instinctive behaviors (see chapter 7). For several genes, we can show that estrogens or progestins can turn on their expression and, in turn, that their gene products play a role in female reproductive behavior (chapter 7). Genes are controlled by proteins called *transcription factors* that bind to their DNA and affect the rate at which their corresponding messenger RNAs are synthesized. The importance of those gene transcription factors, which are hormone receptors, is just now confirmed with gene knockout techniques. That is, simply deleting the gene for one of these hormone receptors has shown how powerful it is in the governance of reproductive behavior (Ogawa et al., 1996; see chapter 7). In addition, a case in which the gene produces enkephalin, a small sequence of five amino acids secreted by neurons and distinguished by opiumlike behavioral effects, demonstrates a fascinating link between sex behavior and pain reduction (Bodnar et al., 1998).

In fact, estrogens can act through their estrogen receptor (a transcription factor) to turn on the gene for the progesterone receptor (another transcription factor) the role of which in a female-typical mating behavior (lordosis behavior) has been demonstrated by three separate technical approaches: (1) by the gene knockout technique; (2) by receptor blockers (such as RU486, now known as *Mifepristone*); and (3) by microinjections into the brain of a DNA sequence—antisense DNA—designed to "foul up" the operation of a specific messenger RNA. Lordosis behavior (treated in detail in chapter 6) is a standing response coupled with a strong vertebral dorsiflexion, typical of female quadrupeds, which allows the male to fertilize. In these lower animals, without lordosis behavior, reproduction will not occur. It turned out to be a well-chosen model for the molecular explanation of behavior because of its motoric simplicity and because its extreme estrogenic and progestigenic dependencies allowed us to bring molecular genetic tools to bear. Altogether, the aforementioned pattern of evidence will prove, for the first time, the role of a specific transcription factor in a specific behavior.

Sometimes, hormonal effects on brain have the capacity to multiply one another. In a small group of hypothalamic neurons, estrogen can enhance the expression of oxytocin, a string of nine amino acids that activates certain smooth muscles and certain neurons, and estrogens also turn on the gene for the oxytocin receptor (see chapter 10). The combined effects on the oxytocin itself and on its receptor should work in the same direction. Actually, they should synergize with each other. Likewise, estrogen facilitates expression of the enkephalin gene (enkephalin being an opioid peptide) and also turns on the gene for the opioid receptor of the delta type through which enkephalin acts uniquely.

We can now reason (see chapters 7 and 9) all the way from molecular genetic and cellular detail to the explanation of how hormones and environment interact to control behavior. Furthermore, these basic cellular mechanisms remain in place in the human brain (see chapter 8). As a result, modern neurobiological, molecular, and behavioral discoveries tell us where, in scientific terms, some of our sexual desires and behaviors originate.

1. SEX DIFFERENCES

We have been exploring the obvious sex differences in reproductive behavior (chapters 5 and 7). The brain mechanisms of such differences, which depend on the early impact of androgenic hormones on the brain, have been confirmed by the antisense DNA technique and by receptor gene knockouts. In XY humans (i.e., genetic males), sex behavior can be reversed following mutations of not only the gene for the androgen receptor (which binds testosterone) but also the gene for an enzyme that metabolizes testosterone.

2. GENES REGULATE BEHAVIOR

Altogether, some of the lessons of gene-behavior relations can now be laid out (chapter 7). Initially, hormone-dependent brain mechanisms led the way toward understanding of these lessons because of the ability of molecular endocrinology to nourish our field of brain research. Among neuroendocrine mechanisms, estrogen-dependent systems have proved to be the easiest to study. Though some of the basic, elementary effects of estrogens on female mating behavior (chapters 5 and 7) allow the demonstration of direct routes of causation from gene to behavior, sexual differentiation and other processes related to reproductive development reveal several indirect routes.

C. Biological Axioms: A Harmony of Mechanisms Satisfy Biological Requirements

Hormonally driven transcription factors interact with one another to control behavior in a manner that appears to satisfy some of the biological requirements for sensible limitations on reproduction. That is, a variety of terrible environmental circumstances should restrain the instinct toward reproduction. The manner in which thyroid hormone receptors, themselves gene transcription factors, interfere with estrogen receptor activities in the brain (chapter 7) seems to provide a mechanism whereby potentially damaging environmental cold or environmental stress would block inappropriate reproductive behavior. More generally, our explorations of hormone-driven transcription factor cooperation and competition appear to open up a new level of neural integration, superimposed on the neuroanatomical, electrophysiological, and neurochemical levels of integration that we neurobiologists know and love. At the end of the day, the symphony of transcription factors must, in principle, satisfy the requirements for biologically adaptive reproduction (see figure 1.2).

Symphony for Body Accompanied by Brain

A *peptide* is a small fragment of a protein that has a recognizable functional effect. A *neuropeptide* is a peptide manufactured by a nerve cell. Oxytocin and other neuropeptides seem to obey a law that the behavioral effects of a neuropeptide in brain will be consonant with its effects elsewhere in the body (see chapter 10). This tendency toward lawfulness first was discovered for the neuropeptide that governs reproductive endocrinology and reproductive behavior: gonadotropin-releasing hormone (GnRH). Nerve cells that produce GnRH undergo a developmental migration that is almost funny: Instead of being born directly in the brain, as other neurons are, they are born in the olfactory pit and must migrate up the nose into the forebrain. As expected from the aforementioned biological axioms, once there, under normal synaptic controls, GnRH-producing neurons work to render mating behavior congruent with the ovarian and testicular physiological and biochemical processes central to reproduction (chapter 10). Even as different organs and different endocrine glands elsewhere in the body participate in driving different instinctive behaviors through hypothalamic neurons, these hypothalamic neurons use distinct anatomical pathways to activate biologically appropriate behaviors (chapter 10).

D. LIBIDO: HUMANS AS ANIMALS

To what extent do these neurobiological themes (analyzed in animal brains) mean anything for human behavior? A lot. Freud's concept of libido covers the most primitive aspects of human desire, explaining the impact of truly physiological forces on feelings and behaviors (chapter 8). Could libido depend on the type of mechanisms we have explored? We can document at least 17 broad domains of sex hormone actions on brain and behavior that truly were conserved as animals evolved toward humans. Thus, to the extent that we have explained mechanisms of sexual behavior and motivation in animals, presumably, we have explained a primitive component of human sex drive: Even as the highest culture-laden aspects of human brain performance—the Apollonian aspects—have evolved greatly from higher animal brains to the human condition, the portions of our feelings given over to the lowest and most primitive desires (the Dionysian) have remained the same, apparently to a humbling extent.

E. MORE GLOBAL EFFECTS OF HORMONES ON BEHAVIOR

Sexual motivation is very fine, both to experience and to explain, but much broader behavioral tendencies and more global aspects of brain function are

---

susceptible to sex hormone influences as well (chapter 10). In their service, oxytocin and vasopressin are both neuropeptides, each composed of only nine amino acids, molecules seemingly quite small for their range of physiological effects. More amazingly, only two of those nine amino acids are different between the two neuropeptides, yet their behavioral actions are most distinct. Oxytocin released in the brain promotes the behaviors of affiliation, whereas vasopressin is associated with stress. Estrogen increases oxytocin secretion and the sensitivity of oxytocin receptors, whereas stress decreases it (chapter 10).

Oxytocin can not just be dumped into a given brain region to achieve a given behavioral effect. Instead, a principle that you might almost expect operates: A neuropeptide's effect on a neural system depends on the amount already released. Further, a lesson which we have found to be true for oxytocin emerges as well: The effect of a neuropeptide depends not only on the genetic background of the animal but on the precise environmental circumstances of the testing (chapter 10).

1. BEYOND SEX: WIDESPREAD EFFECTS ON GROWTH

Trophic actions of hormones in brain tissue are exciting because they link neuroanatomy and neurochemistry to modern developments in cell and molecular biology. Years ago, we found a massive stimulation of growth-related reactions in hypothalamic neurons by long-term estrogenic treatment (chapter 11). The hormone effect was obvious both from ultrastructural measurements and from the amount of ribosomal RNA, a ubiquitous type of RNA constituting part of the cell's "factory" for making new proteins. The estrogen-induced elevation of ribosomal RNA was discovered in so-called molecular hybridization studies using a radioactively labeled probe to measure the amount of ribosomal RNA per neuron.

This type of growth-related hormone action might be important for humans. In subpopulations of women, estrogens can heighten mood, whereas progestins are followed (under some circumstances) by depression and malaise. Both the trophic actions of estrogens and the mood effects have implications for cognitive functions in all humans but especially for aging individuals (chapter 11).

F. SUMMARY

The major questions and topics of the book have been introduced. We will see that the harmony of mechanisms in the service of biologically adaptive reproduction astonishes even the scientist who was prepared to discover them. This harmony is evident at the molecular level (with proved cooperation and competition among transcription factors), at the neurophysiological level (by stimulation of synergistic descending motor control systems), and at the behavioral level (by early hormone-dependent behaviors cascading toward later hormone-dependent behaviors).

For the first time, we are able to reason all the way from molecular genetics and cellular detail to the explanation of how hormones and environmental stimuli interact to control behavior—in this case, specifically motivated sexual responses. Doing so has rendered apparent that human sexual drive may rely also on the same mechanisms as those of higher animals. In this way, our instinctive behaviors are limited by the same physiological imperatives as operate in higher animals and thus are more likely to remain in harmony with objective, biologically important environmental circumstances.

Abraham Maslow knew that higher cognitive abilities could be placed in the service of lower drives (chapter 2). This notion makes sense, because in the well-orchestrated symphony of endocrine, neuronal, and molecular mechanisms portrayed in this book, instinctive behaviors and the motivations associated with them clearly have been geared toward survival and reproduction. After all, if sex behavior were not enjoyable, we might fail to do it.

2

SLAVES OF LOVE?

The third (principle), having many forms, has no special name, but is denoted by the general term "appetitive," from the extraordinary strength and vehemence of the desires of eating and drinking and the other sensual appetites . . . (IX, 581, p. 839)

AND

And are there not many other cases in which we observe that when a man's desires violently prevail over his reason, he reviles himself . . . (IV, 440, p. 703)

YET

Are not necessary pleasures those of which we cannot get rid, and of which the satisfaction is a benefit to us? And they are rightly so, because we are framed by nature to desire both what is beneficial and what is necessary, and cannot help it. (VIII, 559, p. 817)

—*The Dialogues of Plato: The Republic,* trans. B. Jowett

In the movie *Roxanne,* the American comedian Steve Martin plays a small-town fire chief who is skilled and respected as a sensitive and articulate leader. Yet, at different points in this film, he performs dangerous acrobatic ascents and descents of Roxanne's house. Why? Later in this story, based on *Cyrano de Bergerac,* Martin's character displays great self-effacing humor as he enumerates 20 crude jokes about his oversized nose. He even helps a tongue-tied "hunk" to court Roxanne.

What is going on? When you see costar Darryl Hannah, you will be able to guess. The Steve Martin character is serving up a sparkling array of physical and mental accomplishments at the altar of love. That higher human faculties might be placed at the service of lower drives and motivations is not a new idea. What is brand new is that the neurobiological, endocrine, molecular, and behavioral data in this book and the inferences drawn from them explain how one form of motivation works. Neural and genetic facts are drawn into a detailed explanation of one biological form of motivation.

A. HIERARCHIES OF DRIVE

Lower drives must be satisfied before higher drives are addressed. The great psychologist Abraham Maslow (1954) discerned that human beings would not make concerted efforts to satisfy higher levels of drives before lower levels of drives had been fulfilled. Figure 2.1 illustrates in broad form some of the drives about which Maslow talked. Concentrating on calculus is difficult if you are hungry. If you are freezing, you could be distracted from physics. Is microeconomics really that interesting on an evening in which your date is going out with someone else?

Some of the drives in question are controlled by hormones. Hormones are chemicals—usually steroids, proteins or peptides—produced in a bodily organ, circulated in the bloodstream, and acting in a different part of the body. We have been able easily to see how hormones produced in bodily organs outside the brain, coming to the brain, and acting in the brain might control behaviors in a biologically useful way (table 2.1).

Sex behaviors afforded the first examples of success in this field and remain the motivational tendencies whose mechanisms are best understood. Es-

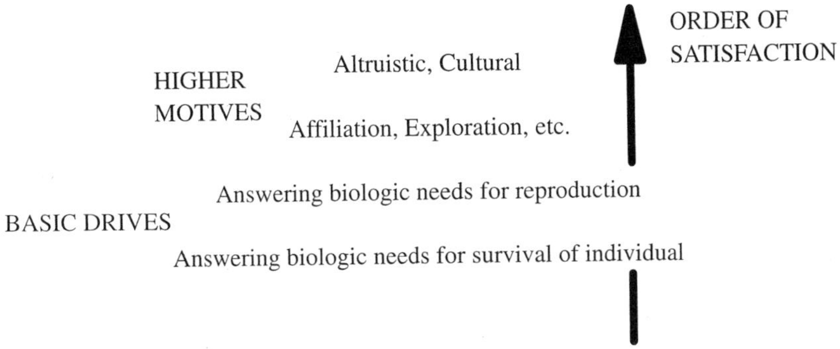

ORDER OF
SATISFACTION

HIGHER   Altruistic, Cultural
MOTIVES
                Affiliation, Exploration, etc.

          Answering biologic needs for reproduction
BASIC DRIVES
          Answering biologic needs for survival of individual

Figure 2.1   Basic drives answering biological needs are satisfied before "higher motives" are addressed. Such higher motives in humans include esthetic preferences, elevation of self-esteem, heightened creativity, and what Maslow termed "self-actualization." (See the work of Abraham Maslow, for example, *Motivation and Personality*, 1954.)

Table 2.1 Some examples of hormone-influenced drives

Organ	Hormone*	Drive state/ Response	Biological use
Ovaries	Estrogen (E)+ Progesterone (P)	Sex/Courtship, Lordosis	Permits fertilization
Testes	Testosterone	Sex/Mounting, copulation	Supplies sperm
Ovaries	Increased estrogen Decreased progesterone	Parental	Cares for young
Adrenal glands	Cortisol Corticosterone	Stress	Protects individual from harm
Fat	Leptin	Satiety	Monitors fat stores
Adrenals	Aldosterone	Salt hunger	Protects body electrolyte–fluid balance
Testes	Testosterone	Aggression	Defends individual and territory

*Hormones effect drive and response by circulating in the blood and entering brain.

trogens and progesterones affecting genetic females particularly and testosterone or its metabolites affecting genetic males in their pursuit of females revealed neural mechanisms worth studying. Consider also, though, maternal behavior, in which high ratios of estrogen to progesterone, identical to those at the end of pregnancy, will foster species-typical parental behaviors. Aggressive behavior can depend also on hormones. Violence by males during courtship is very much influenced by testosterone, whereas in females, maternal aggression during lactational states can be impressive. However, in human beings, testosterone-correlated aggression is a prominent statistical feature of many societies. In domestic violence, a high percentage of the incidents are started by males. Among perpetrators of homicide, the ratio of males to females is large indeed. Even across many societies on the face of this planet, the elevation of homicide rates by males (committed against unrelated males) shoots up at puberty and declines steadily after the high testosterone times of the early twenties.

Testosterone alone is not sufficient for aggression. In fact, in the genetically altered estrogen receptor knockout mouse, we found diminished aggressiveness, indicating that the estrogen receptor in the brain may be a culprit here as well.

Not just sex and aggression but feeding and drinking can be hormone-driven. Estrogens can reduce food intake, as can newly cloned proteinaceous signals coming from fat tissue (for Leptin, see Zhang et al., 1994). Equally obvious are the effects of hormones related to water and salt balance (see table 2.1).

1. BIOLOGICAL HARMONY

In fact, eminent biological sense mandates that the problems of solving lower drives must be addressed before "higher motives" can be considered. After all, one must start with the supposition that behavior is organized to satisfy the axiomatic requirements for survival and reproduction. If these needs are not met, no organism or species can exist to pursue higher aims. If survival-based behaviors are not successful, cultural and esthetic goals cannot be pursued; it simply must be this way. The only sure way to discover new principles about animal brain structure and the control of animal behavior is to start with the obvious, axiomatic biological requirements for survival and reproduction and to reason "geometrically" from there to deduce the behavioral requirements in any particular environmental situation.

2. JURASSIC BRAIN

Can we accurately be portrayed as raging beasts controlled by hormones and other sources of lower drives? Not at all. Even though intellectual accomplishments, physical feats, and various cultural pursuits may be understood with lower drives as base causes, our human culture would not be what it is if lower brain circuitry were not controlled by more sophisticated modern circuits. Together with the evolution of our fine sensory capacities and our skilled muscular limbs, our cultured brains evolved to surround the more primitive aspects

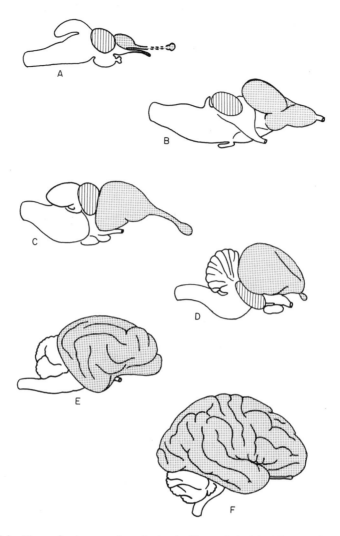

Figure 2.2   Views of various vertebrate brains, looking at their right sides. Vertebrate brains are built around the ventricular system, as taught by the late Professor Walle J.H. Nauta, with typical fish brains closely organized around the ventricles and larger, more sophisticated vertebrate brains surrounding the "periventricular fish" system. This illustration shows the superimposed progressive increase in the relative size of the cerebral hemisphere (stippled area) as we move from codfish (*A*) to frog (*B*) and to alligator (*C*) and then to pigeon (*D*), to cat (*E*), and eventually to human (*F*). These drawings are not to scale and are based on previous illustrations from Strong and Elwyn (1964). The optic tectum (vertical lines) is covered up in the two mammalian brains (*E* and *F*) by the burgeoning cerebral cortex. The cortex (coming from the Latin word for "rind") covers over more primitive brain structures, again illustrating the tendency for the earliest evolved neural systems to be close to the ventricles and for the latest evolved to be wrapped around the outside. (Reproduced from Nauta & Karten, 1970; see source for more detail.)

of our brain (figure 2.2). At the Massachusetts Institute of Technology, our teacher, Professor Walle J.H. Nauta, explained it this way: We have a fish brain inside a reptile brain inside a mammalian brain inside a human brain. So if, with the grossest and most primitive human tendencies in mind, we have been explaining sex drive in a way that corresponds to human sexual libido, in the long run, we hope also to understand the moderating influences imposed by more modern brain circuitry on this lower instinct.

B. SUMMARY

Lower drives can preempt higher drives in their demand for immediate satisfaction. In fact, our higher capacities can be placed in the service of our lower instinctual needs. Moreover, this hierarchy makes good biological sense. How may the detailed neural and molecular mechanisms of instincts and drives be analyzed? Advice: Start simple. Consider Jacques Loeb and his scorpions.

II

Findings and Proofs

Summarizing demonstrations from a large number of neuroanatomical, neuro-physiological, and molecular biological experiments. Together, they form a tight explanation of simple reproductive behaviors and also reveal mechanisms of basic sex drive, including human libido.

3

TROPISMS

. . . the subject of animal conduct can be treated by the quantitative methods of the physicist . . . (p. 7)

The analysis of animal conduct only becomes scientific insofar as it
drops the question of purpose and reduces the reactions of animals
to quantitative laws. (p. 18)

—Jacques Loeb, *Forced Movements, Tropisms & Animal
Conduct,* 1918

The occurrence of learning and memory and the various complexities of behavior require the existence of a set of behavioral responses that can be altered.
Therefore, neurobiologists must answer the most elementary question: Why do
animals or humans do anything at all? Though this question can be tackled for
higher animals (including humans), answers appeared more readily for the simplest of creatures. Enter the pioneer, Jacques Loeb.

The scientist who would bring the systematic study of behavior into the
realm of experimental biology was born Isaak Loeb in the German town of
Mayen in 1859 (Pauly, 1987). During his adolescent years, both his parents

died. Because of his Uncle Harry's interests, Loeb was subjected to a conservative cultural education (figure 3.1) in a "gymnasium" but, bored and arrogant, he broke with that tradition as soon as he graduated. Beginning to study medicine, he encountered some of the early problems of brain physiology at just about the time that the medical profession moved toward assuming a scientific status.

For Loeb, cerebral localization of function held special interest. However, the touchstone for some of his most important contributions to twentieth-century biology came not from the medical faculty but from his contact with a Wurzburg botanist named Julius Sachs. Plants could be manipulated during elegant, technically simple experiments in a manner that higher animals could not. Jacques Loeb's enthusiasm for explaining the simplest reactions of small animals to well-controlled stimuli eventually would feed into an "engineering ideal." He would insist on rigorous experimental answers to the conundrums of the control of behavior.

Moving to the United States, Loeb thrived at the University of California and subsequently was attracted to the Rockefeller Institute, whose scientific director, Simon Flexner, regarded Loeb as a pure research genius in the sphere occupied by Newton, Faraday, and Einstein. Although during his time Loeb elevated the status of a mechanistic biological approach to behavior even to the point of public awareness, his contributions are barely remembered today.

A. JACQUES LOEB'S TROPISMS

One of Loeb's central concerns in his systematic experimentation was to demonstrate the reliability of tropisms: instinctual responses to well-controlled stimuli, shown especially easily in the orientation of animals to bilaterally asymmetrical stimuli. Through simplifying his stimuli, responses, and intellectual concepts, Loeb was trying to avoid the pseudoscientific "metaphysical" thinking of previous scholastic debates and instead to take on a hardheaded "engineering standpoint" in his scientific activity. By doing so, he arrived at prin-

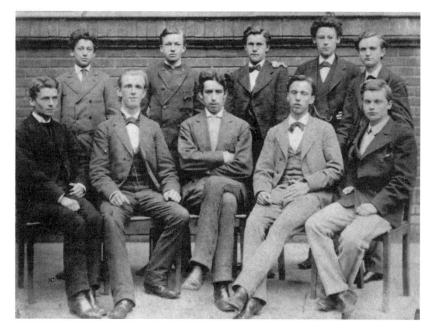

Figure 3.1 Jacques Loeb (seated center front) with schoolmates in Germany at the age of 18. (From Pauly, 1987.)

ciples of animal sensitivity and responsivity that laid the conceptual groundwork for the rigorous study of the biology of motivation.

B. SCORPIONS

Loeb's fascination with the control over the behavior of animals by simple, discoverable stimuli found an illustration in the tendency of certain animals to go toward a source of light (Loeb, 1918). Consider water scorpions (figure 3.2). When a light source is on the animal's right side, the animal breaks bilateral symmetry. The legs on the left side of the body are extended and on the right side are bent (see figure 3.2, top). When instead the light is placed behind the animal, the scorpion's body is raised in front with its head held high in the air (see figure 3.2, bottom). The opposite placement of the light (in front) reverses the animal's response; now the body is lowered, and the head is bent down (see figure 3.2, bottom). Thus is pictured a successful example of Loeb's "behavioral engineering."

C. FLIES

Likewise with flies, Loeb derived a great deal from considerations of symmetry and its laws. For example, he showed that many flies have a tendency to creep upward, oriented in their vertical movement by the downward force of gravity. "When a perfectly symmetrical insect is put on a vertical stick, it walks upward in a straight line" (Loeb, 1918, p. 71). Then, what would happen if stimuli impinging on the animal are rendered asymmetrical? While examining flies in which one eye had been blackened, he noticed that the fly had a tendency to move in circles with the intact eye toward the center, because on one side of the body, the tension of the flexors prevails and, on the other side of the body, the tension of the extensors prevails. As a consequence (figure 3.3), the fly will not move up the vertical stick in a straight line but can only creep in a spiral. Loeb's simplifying, systematic approach to this organism's behavior was rewarded.

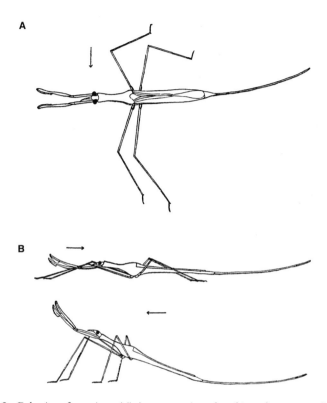

Figure 3.2   Behavior of scorpions. (*A*) Asymmetry introduced into the posture of the water scorpion *Ranatra* when the animal is illuminated from the right side. The legs on the right side of the body are bent, and those on the left side are extended. (Adapted from figure 17 in Loeb, 1918.) (*B*) Alteration in the posture of *Ranatra* according to whether light is in front of the animal (*top*) or behind the animal (*bottom*). (Adapted from figure 18 in Loeb, 1918.)

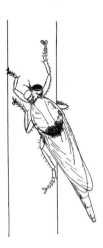

Figure 3.3   Behavior of flies. Loeb (1918, p. 71) noted that many insects put on a vertical stick would walk upward in a straight line. However, with one eye blackened (in his figure 27, the right eye), the fly would creep up the stick in a spiral pattern. (From Loeb, 1918.)

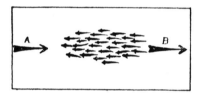

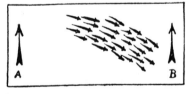 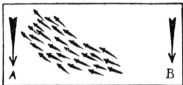

Figure 3.4   Orienting behavior of fish. In this experiment, fish oriented their movements against the direction in which a visual stimulus was moved. (*Top*) Hand movement or striped stimulus movement in the direction of A and B caused them to swim straight forward. (*Bottom left*) Facing toward stimulus B moving to the left, they moved to the right. (*Bottom right*) Facing toward stimulus A moving to the left, they moved to the right. (Adapted from figure 39, p.132 in Loeb, 1918.)

D. FISH

Loeb was interested in a variety of stimuli whose effects on the behavior of lower animals were lawful and predictable. In the case of fish, he quoted the experiments of Garrey, who observed the behavior of sticklebacks, which are "rheotropic." When these fish were kept in an aquarium and a sheet of paper with black stripes was moved constantly in front of the aquarium, the fish oriented themselves against the direction in which the paper and its stripes moved (figure 3.4). Previous experimenters carefully had distinguished the effects of moving retinal images on the fishes' behavior from the possible actions of movement against water (Loeb, 1918). Again, with an entire group of organisms, Loeb successfully illustrated his careful, stepwise approach to behavioral explanation.

E. SUMMARY

In all these examples and in many others, Loeb and subsequent workers could demonstrate experimentally how a particular response came to occur and how it was governed and controlled lawfully. The clarity of Loeb's findings allowed a simple, mechanistic account of complete, "molar" behaviors and depended on his choice of elementary responses in lower organisms. Of course, his success inspired us to search for the optimal mammalian model that had the correct combination of simplicity in its performance and regulation on the one hand and potentially important principles of neuronal and molecular integration on the other hand. Loeb's animals' responses had no trace of a motivational component; in any case, these lower animals had both a very limited capacity to sense stimuli and an impoverished repertoire of responses. What can be said about the greater flexibility of behavioral responses in higher organisms having more choices?

4

The Concept of Drive

From the brain, and from the brain only, arise our pleasures, joys . . .

—Hippocrates, *The Sacred Disease,* trans. W.H.S. Jones

The concept of drive can be treated simply and strictly as having a solid logical role in the neural explanation of changes in behavior; however, motivational concepts applied in human life take on a variety of shadings as complex as the human mind itself. Not all are limited to reproductive or ingestive behaviors or to commodities for human comfort. In his recent book *Emotional Intelligence,* Dan Goleman illustrates how positive motivational states can lead to a wide variety of practices which effectively make us behave as more intelligent human beings. With this point of view, he amplifies one aspect of what we already learned from Howard Gardner's book, *Frames of Mind.* In this and subsequent books, Gardner shows that high intelligence comes not solely from literary, logical, or mathematical ability but is manifest in at least seven different domains of life. Logically, from that concept follows the idea that highly intelligent performance is not just for quick thinkers and deep philosophers. Therefore, even for human cognitive accomplishments far beyond simple animal instinctive responses, motivation counts.

A. Logical Need for Motivational Concepts

Concepts of drive or motivation are necessary to explain the appearance of animals' or human beings' goal-directed responses due to changes in bodily state, such as hunger, thirst, or sex hormones.

Consider a higher animal or a human being in a basal state. Present a well-defined stimulus (S1) and notice the absence of a specific response (R1). Then change something in that animal or human being—perhaps making the animal hungry or imposing a hormonal change. Finally, perhaps the next day, at the same time of day, with the animal essentially the same age and given the same weather and the same environment and the like, present that well-defined stimulus (S1) again and now notice the *presence* of the response (R1). How do we explain this form of neuroplasticity (i.e., this type of functional change in the central nervous system)? We must have a concept for what was changed in the animal; particularly for the type of example given, the concepts of drive (motivation) have served well (figure 4.1).

B. Criteria for Proof (Illustrated)

Given the logical necessity of motivational concepts, how do experimental biologists study their properties? Any individual experimental result might be interpreted in a variety of ways, and the properties of motivational changes could be confused with other physiological and neuronal adaptations. The answer to this problem is to use *convergent operations*. That is, when an entire variety of means are used for increasing or decreasing the motivation and a variety of responses are used similarly for assessing the amount of motivation (both instinctive consummatory responses and learned responses) and if all the stimulus-response relationships come out as predicted, the scientific usefulness of that particular concept of motivation is ensured. As an obvious example, the motivational validity of thirst is proved by a variety of manipulations. They could include rendering the animal water-deprived; predrinking by mouth; injection; reduction by a stomach fistula; and the like, followed by a variety of response measures:

	Trial 1		Trial 2
Fixed Stimulus (sweet taste)	Presented to tongue		same
Environment	constant		same
Age	constant		same
t of day	fixed		same
t of year	fixed		same
Internal change	satiated	Δ	food deprived
Response	**None**	Δ	**strong positive response**

Δ

DEDUCE ⦂   **MOTIVATION**

Figure 4.1   If between two presentations of a stimulus held physically constant a variety of conditions are also held constant but the response changes, logic requires the inference that an "intervening variable" (namely the level of *motivation*) also has changed. The change in motivation explains the change in behavioral response.

amount of fluid consumed, approach responses to the water, and learned responses motivated by the need for water (Miller, 1959, 1967; Pfaff, 1982). Even as the concepts of physical science have proved useful and convincing because of their generality, as confirmed in functional equations, such biological concepts as motivation are proved scientifically useful because of their explanatory power with respect to a variety of stimulus-response relationships.

A long list of biologically based motivations observed in animal and human behavior has been characterized in this way. Some motivations are clearly homeostatic (i.e., necessary for proper physiological balance within the individual). Hunger, thirst, salt hunger, and maintenance of a proper core body temperature are among them. Others, such as maintenance of body temperature and the reduction of pain, also are necessary for the survival of the individual. Some, such as an exploratory drive or a need for mastery, have been demonstrated repeatedly in animal and human behavior, although their biological justifications are more subtle. The need for sleep is obvious, but analysis of sleep has fallen more into the province of circadian rhythm studies than of motivational theory. Still other motivational systems are connected more closely to the preservation of the species: masculine sexual behavior, feminine sexual behavior, and maternal behavior are examples.

Among these motivational systems, some hormone-influenced drives already were mentioned in chapter 2. Comparing and contrasting all those that have proved favorable for analysis of neural mechanisms—male sexual behavior, female sexual behavior, maternal behavior, and salt hunger—is easy (table 4.1). For example, the importance of mineralocorticoid hormones, steroids such as aldosterone produced by the adrenal gland, for salt hunger has been documented (Fluharty & Sakai, 1995; Sakai et al., 1986). Blocking gene expression for the receptor in the brain that mediates adrenal steroid hormone effects on salt appetite will reduce the amount of salt ingested (Sakai et al., 1996). In fact, these hormonal effects on salt hunger interact with gender (Chow et al., 1992) and with estrogen administration (Jonkalass & Buggy, 1984, 1985; Kisley et al., 1998). Females ingest more saline per day than do males, perhaps because of the effects of estrogens on brain peptide hormone receptors. Overall, the neu-

Table 4.1 Some hormone–dependent drives in animals

	Female Sex	Male Sex	Maternal (parental)	Salt Hunger	Aggression
Biological need	Reproduction	Reproduction	Reproduction	Homeostatic	Defense of individual or territory
Hormone	E and progestins	Androgens	E and dropping P	Aldosterone	Androgens
Site of action	Hypothalamus	Preoptic area	Preoptic area	Amygdala	?
Hormone receptor	ER,PR	AR,ER	ER,PR	MR	AR,ER★
Stimulus	Somatosensory	Odor, vision, touch	Odor, sound, touch	Salty taste	Attacker
Response	Lordosis	Mount and intromission	Retrieve, crouch	Ingest	Box, wrestle, bite
Result	Fertilization	Fertilization	Young survive	Maintain salt-water balance	Individual survives or reproduces

E, estrogen; P, progesterone; ER, estrogen receptors; PR, progesterone receptors; AR, androgen receptors; MR, mineralocorticoid receptors.
★ER gene–deficient mice do not attack (Ogawa et al., 1997).

roendocrinology and molecular endocrinology of steroid sex hormones and their receptors have allowed the deepest and most extensive research progress. Therefore, this book can make its best points in the neuronal systems related to sex (chapters 5 and 7).

C. TWO-COMPONENT THEORY OF DRIVE

Classic research on motivational behavior by Hull, Neal Miller, Bolles, and their colleagues showed that every drive has two components: a generalized drive common to all forms of motivation and a specific component dependent on particular biological needs and leading to specific behaviors that reduce the needs (figure 4.2). Such a two-component theory of biological drives maps onto classic distinctions of the functions of motivation, which are both to *energize* behavior and to *direct* behavior. In turn, for lordosis behavior, these biological and behavioral functions of drive map nicely onto a known neural circuit (see chapter 6).

The *activating* functions of drive surely depend on the reticular core of the brain, namely the classic ascending reticular activating system described by Giovanni Moruzzi from Pisa and Horace Magoun at the University of California at Los Angeles. The ascending reticular activating system alerts (excites, "wakes up") neural systems widespread in the forebrain on receipt of sudden, disturbing, stressful, or painful stimuli. Involving several transmitters and multiple neuronal pathways, the ascending reticular activating system first was understood through electrophysiological and anatomical techniques. The neuroanatomy and histochemistry of these ascending arousal systems were elucidated brilliantly by a group of Swedish neuroanatomists (Dahlstrom & Fuxe, 1964; Fuxe et al., 1965, 1968, 1970; Hokfelt, 1966, 1967a,b, 1968, 1969; Hokfelt et al., 1974), who discovered with breathtaking virtuosity that noradrenergic and dopaminergic cells in the brainstem give rise to a vast set of ascending projections.

The locus coeruleus clearly plays an important part in this system (Aston-Jones & Valentino, 1996). In recent years, however, the ascending reticular activating system has been subdivided neuroanatomically, neurochemically, and

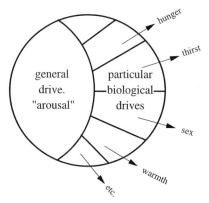

Figure 4.2 Drives, or motivations, have at least two types of components. First is a component necessary for the *energization* of behavior—arousal—that is general across motivational states. Second is mechanisms that respond to humoral and other particular physiological signals arising from specific biological needs, such as hunger, thirst, sex hormones, temperature changes, and the like. This second type of component gives *direction* to motivated behavior.

functionally (Robbins & Everitt, 1996). Importantly, estrogens can influence brainstem noradrenergic neurons, because many, especially in the hindbrain, contain estrogen receptors (Herbison & Simonian, 1996). Through adrenergic projections to the hypothalamus (see data on α_1 receptors in chapter 6) and pre-optic area, this portion of the estrogen effect in brain yields a female aroused, ready to locomote (for courtship and approach responses), muscularly taut, and ready to support the weight of the male (for lordosis behavior).

In contrast, the *particular* features of different biologically driven need states, which *direct* behavior, are represented separately by particular physiological signals to separate limbic forebrain and hypothalamic circuits (figure 4.3). Though the arousal systems discovered by Fuxe, Hokfelt, and their colleagues may be similar across different motivational systems, apparently the mechanisms by which different biologically important need states are represented in fore-brain and hypothalamic neurons are not the same (see figure 4.3; Pfaff, 1982).

Even in the simplest aspects of female reproductive behavior, hormone-sensitive drive states manifest themselves in at least three forms of behavior: instrumental, appetitive, and consummatory. Regarding *instrumental responses,* Professor James Matthews, of New York University, and the author have determined that female rats will learn experimenter-chosen, arbitrarily defined responses to gain access to the male (figure 4.4). Ample evidence (reviewed by Meyerson & Lindstrom, 1971) has been presented to document the hormone sensitivity of female rats' approach responses. *Appetitive responses* too have been illustrated in the rat. Progesterone administration after estrogen priming impressively enhances the female rat's performance of bizarre courtship behaviors (hopping, darting, and head wiggling) that at once demonstrate an extraordinary tautness in all the axial muscles (neck and trunk muscles) of the body (see chapter 6) and serve to draw the male to the female with both partners in their correct positions for copulation. Finally, *consummatory responses,* in the form of lordosis behavior by the female, which permits penetration and fertilization by the male, have been elucidated. The female response is so hormone-dependent (chapter 5) and so simple that its neural circuit could be discovered (chapter 6), the first for a vertebrate animal's behavior.

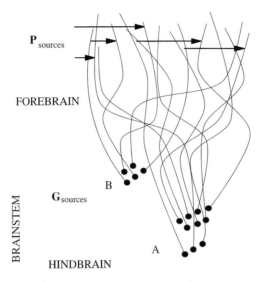

Figure 4.3 Neuroanatomy of two-component drives. As discovered at the Karolinska Institutet during the 1960s, groups of noradrenergic neurons (A) and dopaminergic neurons (B)
located in the hindbrain and midbrain give rise to widely distributed axonal trajectories and
terminations in the forebrain. Excitation and activity of such neurons are likely to comprise
the mechanisms of generalized drive states (G sources). Their concerted actions are at the basis
of electrophysiological and behavioral arousal, the general component of drive. By comparison, for the particular sources (P) of activation of particular drives serving individual biological needs, humoral stimuli, including hormones, act at specific forebrain locations. In each
case, their specific actions determine individualized motivational states. Together, the effect
of generalized arousal (G) and particular biological need states (P) energize and direct motivated behaviors.

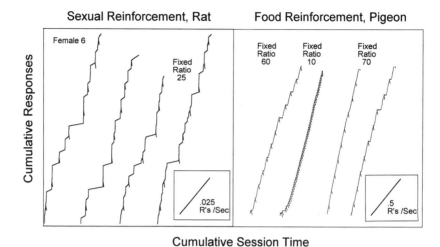

Cumulative Session Time

Figure 4.4   Female rats would learn an arbitrarily chosen response (in this case, pressing on a sensitive button with their noses) to gain access to a stud male rat, thus demonstrating motivation to approach that male. The quantitative characteristics of the behavioral manifestation of this sexual motivation are significantly different from those customary for food reinforcement, for example in the pigeon (food reinforcement data from Ferster & Skinner, 1957). In contrast to food reinforcement, behavioral responses by the female for sexual reinforcement were very slow and did not show the same postreinforcement "scalloping" usually seen after food reward. (Data from Matthews et al., 1997.)

D. SUMMARY

Motivational concepts are required logically to explain the activation and guidance of behavior, including those responses that reflect primitive, biologically based needs. Mechanisms in the brain serving various forms of motivation could be illustrated. However, the greatest progress has been made with hormone-controlled drives, largely because hormonally controlled sex behaviors have submitted easily to detailed neural and molecular-genetic analyses.

5

HORMONE-CONTROLLED DRIVES

Love can do all but raise the Dead.

—Emily Dickinson, "1731"

Luckily for neuroscientists, steroid sex hormones are small, fat-soluble molecules that readily cross the barrier between the blood and the brain and then diffuse freely throughout the brain. After being secreted by the ovaries, testes, and adrenal glands into the blood, the estrogens, androgens, and progestins can flood the brain and, in doing so, they can influence a broad range of behaviors associated with reproduction.

Modern work has delved deeply into those aspects of sex hormone action that depend on the long-term binding of hormones to specific receptors in the cell nucleus. After the transport of the hormone bound to its receptor next to the surface of DNA, specific genes can be turned on. Subsequently, neurons grow and change their chemical and electrical properties. We have demonstrated how these alterations by hormones permit specific reproductive behaviors.

Experiments with infrahuman animals prove that the steroid hormones from sex organs awaken the brain to drive sexual behaviors that otherwise would not have occurred (Beach, 1948; Pfaff et al., 1984). Is this true of humans too?

Among all higher primates, female sexual behavior was thought to be absolutely independent of hormones. Now we know that under some conditions, some fluctuations are detectable according to hormonal state in women. Referred to, in such statements, would not be the most culturally elevated manifestations of romance but rather those primitive urges more akin to lust. These urges have been described most graphically over the years by psychologists, ethologists, and psychoanalysts. However, solid physiological data are obtained much more easily in subhuman primates, such as monkeys. Make no mistake about it: Female monkeys can display courtship and sexual behaviors in the absence of ovarian sex hormones. Nevertheless, discovered among female rhesus monkeys (Bonsall et al., 1978; Michael & Bonsall, 1977; Michael & Zumpe, 1970; Zumpe & Michael, 1970) are clear interactions between the female rhesus monkey's social history and estrogen levels, which determine the probability of her willingness to mate (reviewed by Tannenbaum & Wallen, 1997; Wallen, 1996; Wallen & Tannenbaum, 1997). The human male's mating instincts even more obviously depend on circulating steroids than do women's. That is the best of it: As noted in chapter 2, various forms of violence among human beings also appear to be fostered by testosterone or its metabolites.

These issues of the physiology of lust (as described behaviorally by ethologists, psychologists, and psychoanalysts) increasingly will be socially important. As the "baby boomers" in America, Europe, and Japan enter the new century, the question of the survival of feminine sexuality and masculine mating drives during the aging process will become very prominent (see chapter 11 also).

For the present purpose and for the deepest analysis of neural and molecular mechanisms, it is necessary to figure out how a simple mating behavior works, in terms of central neural mechanisms.

A. SEX HORMONE EFFECTS IN ANIMALS AND HUMANS

Saying that "hormones control behaviors" would be incorrect. Instead, we see that hormones as internal signals have molecular sequelae that *interact* with synaptic inputs from external stimuli to control behavior. In the case of a simple behavior, such as female rat reproductive responses, both the proof of these interactions and their mechanisms have become clear. For example, estrogen administration lowers the threshold for somatosensory stimuli to trigger lordosis behavior (figure 5.1). The neural explanation of how this occurs is manifest in the circuitry summarized in chapter 6.

The overall patterns of sex hormone and sex behavior relationships are remarkably parallel between mammals used for experimental neurobiology and human beings (table 5.1). *In males, the absence of testicular hormones and, in females the long-term absence of ovarian hormones are associated with reduction in sex drive.* With respect to hormone replacement, in males of a wide variety of species, testosterone restores sex drive (Kelley & Pfaff, 1978). Eunuchs do not mate; the harem was safe with them. In fact, men who are criminal sex offenders often crave their antiandrogenic compounds as medical treatment because, to conform to society's rules, they want their dangerously high levels of libido reduced. Likewise, among animals used for experiments, estrogens followed by progestins reliably facilitate mating behavior (e.g., lordosis behavior). In human females, long-term absence of ovarian hormones (as before puberty and after menopause) commonly is associated with reduced sex drive. Surprisingly, androgens followed by progesterone can be effective for increasing sex behavior in females, both in experimental animals (Pfaff, 1970) and in women (Davis & Berger, 1996).

In lower experimental animals, relatively simple stimuli can trigger mating responses if the enormous facilitating actions of steroid sex hormones are present (figure 5.2). Regarding observations among women, the data are largely correlational. Moreover, with our impressive sensory, motor, and intellectual capacities and with our substantial cerebral cortices in gear, we humans are so very subject to a wide variety of cultural and other environmental influences that, quantitatively, sex hormones have a lesser role to play.

From a mechanistic point of view, even though explaining sex behaviors themselves has proved easiest, hormone effects by no means are limited to these responses. In lower animals and humans, both males and females will perform a wide variety of learned responses to gain access to members of the opposite

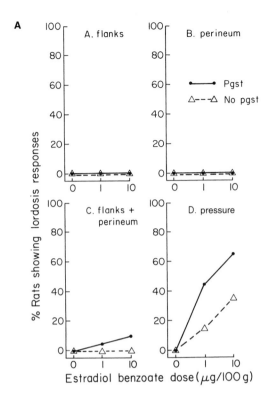

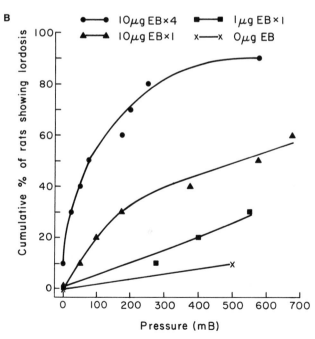

gender. How many college boys and girls have done truly ridiculous things to get next to each other on weekends? In female rats, a long history of research demonstrated that they would perform arbitrary responses or suffer punishment to gain access to the male rat and that, in turn, was facilitated by estrogens (reviewed in Pfaff, 1982). As a recent example, Professor Jim Matthews and the author (as mentioned) (see figure 4.4) saw that female rats will perform any of three arbitrarily chosen responses to gain access to a chamber wherein a stud male rat was housed. Some, but not all, aspects of the female rat's performance are facilitated by estrogens (figure 5.3).

B. PRINCIPLES OF HORMONE ACTIONS ON BEHAVIOR

First, the assertion of efficacy: As noted above, in a wide variety of vertebrate animals, steroid sex hormones work through specific neuronal groups and promote behaviors associated with mating. (See Kelley & Pfaff, 1978, and Meisel & Sachs, 1994, as reviews for males; Pfaff, 1980, contains a review for females.)

Second, for stimulating behavior and for facilitating pituitary hormone release, the *rates of onset* of hormone treatment, the durations, and other temporal features of hormone administration are important (figure 5.4). In males, androgens must be circulating at high levels for long periods to be effective. In females, estrogens are never absent, and their effects seem to build up, working through fast mechanisms, medium-speed mechanisms, and very slow "priming mechanisms" to achieve their overall results (figure 5.5). In contrast, a rapid increase in

Figure 5.1   Interaction of sensory and hormonal inputs to determine female rat reproductive behavior. (*A*) Light cutaneous stimuli applied to the flanks alone (*upper left*), to the perineum alone (*upper right*) or flanks plus perineum (*lower left*) did not trigger lordosis behavior, regardless of estradiol or progesterone treatment. However, cutaneous stimulation of the flanks followed by pressure to the perineum (*lower right*) triggered lordosis behavior to an extent codetermined by the dose of estradiol, especially if supplemented by progesterone. (From Pfaff et al., 1977.) (*B*) The amount of lordosis behavior displayed was an orderly function of the amount of pressure applied to the skin of the perineum of the female rat, the effect of which was magnified according to the dose of estradiol benzoid (EB) with which the female had been treated. (From Kow et al., 1979.)

Table 5.1   Sexual motivation during absence or presence of gonadal hormones in animals and humans

	Behavior of Females					Behavior of Males	
	Ovarian cycle	Ovarian hormones absent	Hormone replacement			Castration	Hormone replacement
			E	E + P	T + P		
Animals	Behavior coordinated with ovulation	None	Present	Maximal	Present	Virtually absent	Mating behavior restored
Humans	Cycling effect not strong	Low (prepubertal) (old age)	Elevated		Elevated*	Virtually absent (e.g., eunuchs, Kallmann's syndrome)	T heightens sex drive

E, estrogen; P, progestins; T, testosterone.
*According to Davis & Burger, 1996. Most clinical results have alternative interpretations.

Causes of sex drive

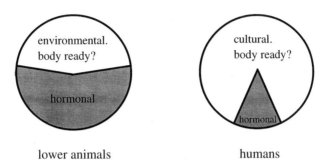

Figure 5.2   Each circle represents 100% of the causes of sex drive in lower animals (*left*) or humans (*right*). In lower animals, steroid sex hormones account for a large part of the determination of sex drive and subsequent mating responses. In addition, animals must sense appropriate stimuli from an adequate mating partner and must receive physiological signals that environmental circumstances permit biologically adaptive mating. In humans, steroid sex hormones account for a relatively smaller portion of sex drive. Other determinants include not only physiological signals from the rest of the body but a wide variety of cultural restraints.

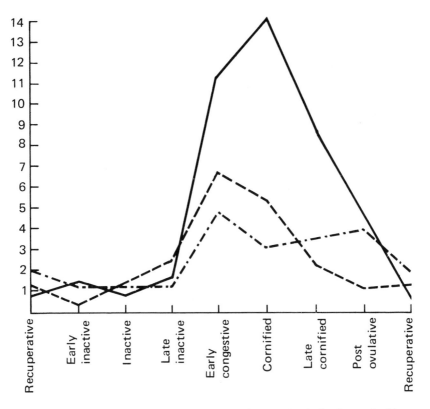

Figure 5.3 Estrogenic hormones can heighten sexual motivation in female rats. In this experiment, typical of a large number of studies (reviewed in Pfaff, 1982), Warner (1927) set up a situation in which female rats had to cross an electric grid to achieve contact with a male rat. The number of times female rats were willing to cross that electric grid (solid line) was greatest at or near the time that the vaginal smear was cornified (Warner, 1927). This histological characteristic of the vaginal smear reflects high levels of natural estrogens circulating in the blood.

Females

Males

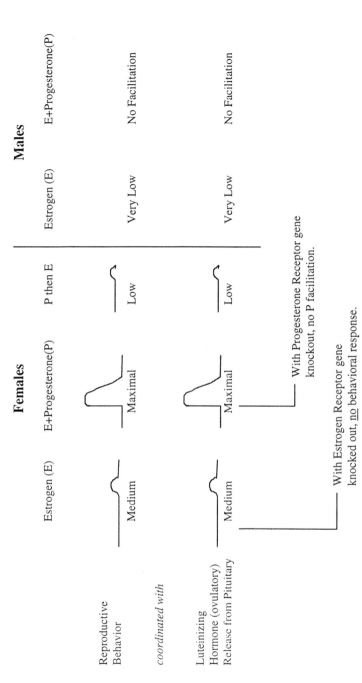

	Estrogen (E)	E+Progesterone(P)	P then E	Estrogen (E)	E+Progesterone(P)
Reproductive Behavior	Medium	Maximal	Low	Very Low	No Facilitation
coordinated with					
Luteinizing Hormone (ovulatory) Release from Pituitary	Medium	Maximal	Low	Very Low	No Facilitation

With Estrogen Receptor gene knocked out, no behavioral response.

With Progesterone Receptor gene knockout, no P facilitation.

Figure 5.4   Reproductive behavioral motivation in the female is coordinated by the concerted actions of estrogens and progestins with the ovulatory luteinizing hormone (LH) release from the pituitary. A short schedule of estrogen treatment can lead to discernible rises in behavior and in LH release. In the female, both behavior and LH release are facilitated massively by a *subsequent* progesterone treatment. Ideally, progesterone follows estrogen by some 48 hours. If instead progesterone is given before estrogen or simultaneously with it, not only will the estrogen effect be blunted but the female is rendered insensitive to subsequent progesterone treatment. There is a large sex difference: Males do not show substantial lordosis behavior or surges of LH. As regards requirement for gene expression, with the estrogen receptor gene knocked out, no lordosis behavior occurs in response to estradiol (Ogawa et al., 1996b). With the progesterone receptor gene knocked out, no facilitatory response occurs after progesterone (Lydon et al., 1995; Ogawa et al., submitted).

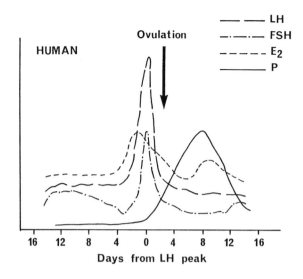

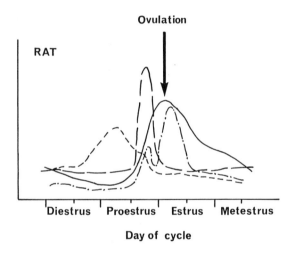

Figure 5.5   Patterns of changes in blood levels of steroid sex hormones (E2, estradiol; P, progesterone) and gonadotropin hormones (LH, luteinizing hormone; FSH, follicle-stimulating hormone) during the human menstrual cycle *(top)* and the rat estrous cycle *(bottom)*. In the female rat, the rise in estradiol followed by the initial elevation in progesterone triggers the ovulatory surge in LH, beautifully coordinated with female reproductive behavior. The synchrony of ovulation with lordosis behavior permits fertilization by the male and subsequent pregnancy. Among women, the tendency is higher libido around the time of ovulation, but hormonal control over this aspect of behavior is not nearly as powerful as in lower animals. The rat data, summarized from the work of George Fink (1977), is in substantial agreement with the work of Butcher et al. (1974) and Smith et al. (1975). The human data have been summarized from the work of Midgley and Jaffe (1986), Ross et al. (1970), Wide et al. (1973), and Keye et al. (1973).

progesterone will facilitate both female reproductive behavior and the ovulatory release of luteinizing hormone (LH) from the pituitary (see figure 5.4), but a longer duration of progesterone action without a sudden increase in this hormone will inhibit both lordosis behavior and the ovulatory release of LH from the pituitary (see figure 5.4; figure 5.6). Amazingly, some actions of estrogens formerly thought to require continuous estrogen presence can be achieved also by brief pulses of estrogen (Parsons et al., 1981, 1982). This type of data gathered in experiments with infrahuman animals may be important for hormone replacement therapy in older women. More to the point, this striking confluence of the temporal requirements for hormone treatments between female rat reproductive behaviors on one hand and ovulation on the other helps to synchronize the two functions: to guarantee that the female will engage in such behavior only when she is ready to ovulate. In such a case, the coordination of endocrine and behavioral events is perfect.

Not only the presence and the duration of hormone treatment but the *order of appearance* of hormones in the brain can be important for stimulating reproductive behavior. Progesterone by itself will not do much but, after a long period of estrogen exposure—at least 24 hours and preferably 48 or 72 hours—progesterone can greatly amplify the effect of estrogen on female-typical behaviors and LH (see figures 5.4 and 5.6). As is seen in chapter 7, gene expression for the progesterone receptor is required for this effect. Gene knockout data, antisense DNA data, and progesterone receptor blocker data all agree on this point.

Finally, when the steroid sex hormones themselves are injected or otherwise administered, their *metabolites* also can be important for triggering reproductive behavior. Testosterone can act in its own chemical form but also can be converted to dihydrotesterone or even (by a different chemical reaction) to estradiol (figure 5.7). The stereotype that estrogens are active only in females and androgens only in males is incorrect. In the genetic male, estrogens actually can help to carry out the mission of androgenic hormones after the chemical conversion just mentioned. On the other side of the coin, in females, androgenic hormones coming from the female's adrenal glands can have important behavioral effects.

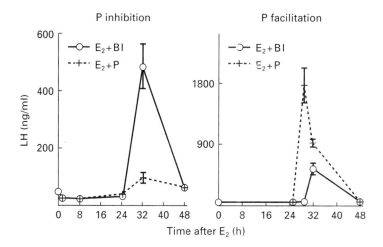

Figure 5.6 When progesterone treatment (P) follows estrogen priming (E2) by 24 hours, progesterone markedly *facilitates* luteinizing hormone release as compared to estrogen priming followed by a blank capsule control (B1, *right*). In contrast, if progesterone is given prior to or concomitantly with estrogen treatment, the progesterone not only *inhibits* robust responses to estrogen (*left*) but renders the female unresponsive to subsequent progesterone facilitation. (From Attardi et al., 1997.)

Figure 5.7 As shown by this pattern of testosterone metabolism, testosterone can act simply as an androgen and also can be metabolized to estradiol. The percentages give estimates of conversion rates in humans. (From Horton, 1989.)

Richard Michael, Doris Zumpe, and their collaborators at Emory University were among a group of investigators who showed that in female primates, adrenal androgens could promote reproductive behaviors. In a completely different way, with an emphasis on steroid biochemistry, the case of progesterone is similarly complicated. Progesterone itself can operate through the progesterone receptor that goes into the nerve cell's nucleus and affects gene expression. When metabolized, progesterone can operate in the brain by affecting transmission through cell membrane receptors for an inhibitory transmitter, GABA.

In summary, the universally important influences of sex steroid hormones on reproductive behaviors involve the specific timing of hormone administration, the order of administration of different hormones, and the chemical modification of these hormones.

C. HORMONE-SENSITIVE NEURONS IN THE BRAINS OF VERTEBRATES

The first studies to pinpoint the precise locations of nerve cells sensitive to sex hormones used a special histochemical hormone-binding technique, hormone receptor autoradiography, in which tritiated estrogen or androgen retained in the nerve cell body and even in the cell nucleus would make its presence known because its very weak β particle was registered in a highly sensitive nuclear track emulsion (Pfaff, 1968a,b). By and large, the results of these hormone-binding studies were confirmed in their neuroanatomical detail by immunocytochemistry for sex hormone receptor protein and, more recently, by in situ hybridization in which gene expression for estrogen receptor or progesterone receptor was charted and shown to be physiologically regulated (Lauber et al., 1990b, 1991a,b; Romano et al., 1989a). Consequently, all these studies are summarized together, as follows.

The major finding was that even though lipid-soluble steroid hormones could cross the blood-brain barrier and, indeed, flood the entire central nervous system, they were retained specifically only in a system of limbic and hypothalamic neurons. In all vertebrate species studied (figures 5.8 and 5.9), sex hormone-binding neuronal groups include, in the telencephalon, the medial amygdala or its homologous structure; the lateral septum or its homologous structure; and the medial preoptic area and the bed nucleus of the stria terminalis. In the hypothalamus, they always comprise the tuberal (or infundibular) cell groups immediately surrounding the pituitary stalk. In the rat, they would be designated the ventral medial nucleus of the hypothalamus, the arcuate nucleus, and the ventral premammillary nucleus (Pfaff & Keiner, 1973). Most exciting was the compilation of neuroanatomical connectivity studies (figures 5.10 through 5.12) showing that these limbic and hypothalamic cell groups share a remarkable degree of interconnection, which suggests that they can indeed act as a physiologically integrated system (Cottingham & Pfaff, 1986; Pfaff & Keiner, 1973). In all vertebrates studied, these forebrain cell groups obviously are involved in the coordinated controls of mating behavior and pituitary gonadotropin release.

In addition to the vertebrate-wide pattern of sex hormone–binding neurons (see figure 5.9) some individual species possess additional sex hormone–binding groups that, in the large majority of cases, turn out to be related to the control of sex hormone–dependent behavior or gonadotropin release. For example, male song birds whose singing is androgen-dependent have androgen-binding neurons in their song control cell groups, as discovered by Zigmond et

Figures 5.8–5.12   Discovery of the exact positions and connections of estrogen-binding neurons in rodent brains led to the characterization of a basic sex hormone-binding limbic-hypothalamic system prominent in the brains of all vertebrates.

Figure 5.8   Estrogen-binding neurons. Five of the transverse levels of an atlas of estrogen-binding neurons in the rat brain. First reported in 1965 (Pfaff, 1965), quantified in 1968 (1968), and replicated and published in greatest topographical detail in 1973 (Pfaff & Keiner, 1973), this atlas pinpointed the locations of neurons with nuclear hormone receptors that bound and retained estrogens. As such, these neurons could be important for mediating the effects either of the classic estrogen receptor or of estrogen receptor-β (Kuiper et al., 1996). Exact locations of estrogen binding neurons are shown as black dots plotted on a rat brain atlas. Where the locations are so dense that individual dots overlapped each other, that subregion is blackened. The neurons in this limbic-hypothalamic system have proved crucial for neuroendocrine and behavioral controls.

———

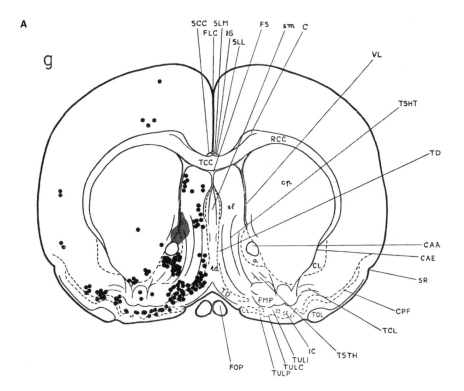

A

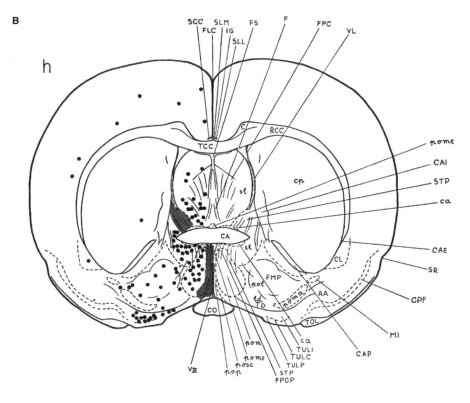

B

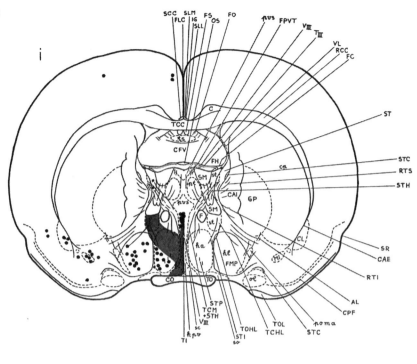

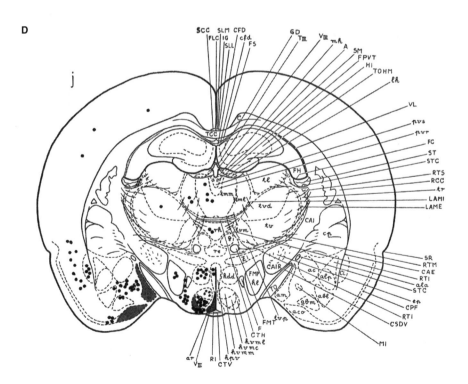

E

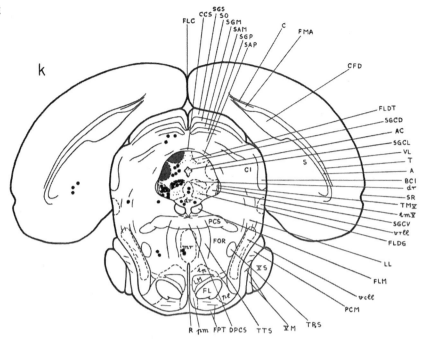

k

SGS
CCS SO
FLC SGM
SAM
SGP
SAP
c FMA
CFD
FLDT
SGCD
AC
SGCL
VL
T
A
BCI
dr
SR
TMⅤ
ℓmⅤ
SGCV
vrℓℓ
FLDG
LL
FLM
vcℓℓ
PCM
CI S
nr
ℓn
M
FL nℓ
PCS
FOR
ⅤS
TRS
ⅤM
R nm FPT DPCS TTS

F

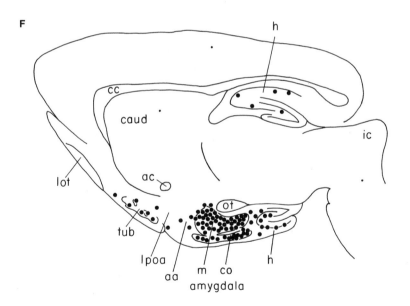

h
cc
caud
ic
lot
ac
tub
lpoa
aa m co
amygdala
h
ot

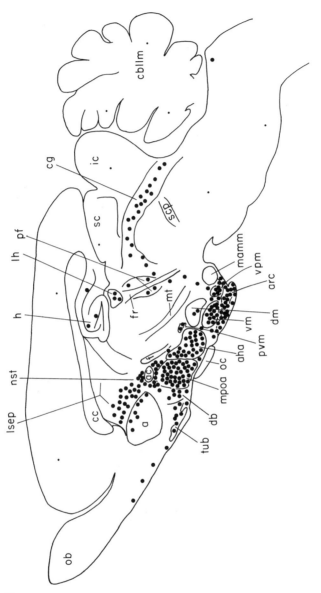

G

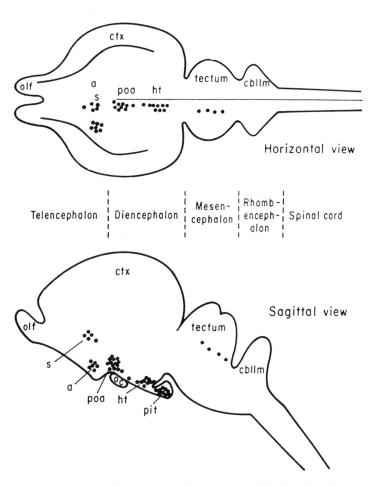

Figure 5.9   Representation for all vertebrate brains. By use of the depiction of a generalized vertebrate brain drawn by Nauta and Karten (1970), the locations of nerve cell groups with high numbers of estrogen-binding neurons are shown as large black dots. Included are the tuberal hypothalamic cell groups, the medial preoptic area, the medial nucleus of the amygdala, and the lateral portion of the septum (first summarized in Morrell & Pfaff, 1978).

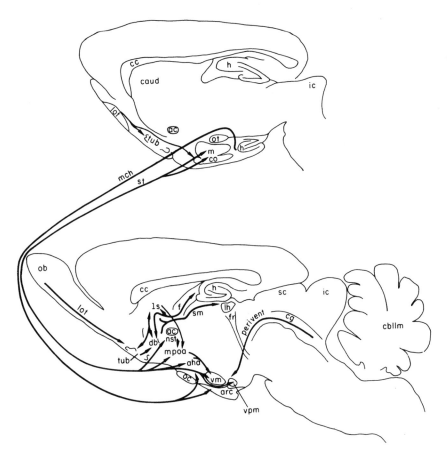

Figure 5.10   Connections in a hormone-responsive neuronal system. For convenience, the top drawing is a schematic depiction of estrogen-binding neuronal groups in sagittal section. The bottom drawing shows the connections already known among those groups in 1973 (Pfaff & Keiner, 1973). Much greater detail was added within an additional decade of neuroanatomical discoveries (Cottingham & Pfaff, 1986) Estrogen-binding neuronal groups tend to project preferentially to other estrogen-binding neuronal groups. The opportunities for neuroendocrine integration and amplification are clear.

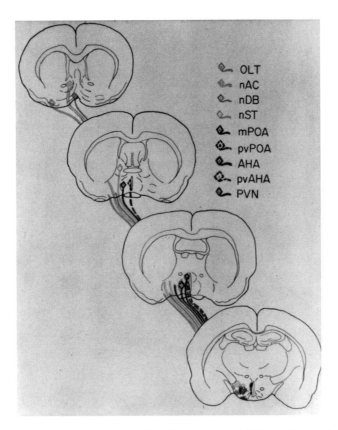

Figure 5.11   For a color reproduction of this figure, see plate 1. Efferents from the basal fore-brain and anterior hypothalamus follow more orderly trajectories than had been anticipated. Axons descending from the olfactory tubercle (OLT), nucleus accumbens (NAC), nuclei of the diagonal band of Broca (NDB), nucleus of the stria terminalis (NST), medial preoptic area (MPOA), periventricular POA (PVPOA), anterior hypothalamic area (AHA), periventricular anterior hypothalamic area (PVAHA), and periventricular nucleus (PVN), have trajectories that approximate "laminar flow" (first published in Pfaff & Conrad, 1978).

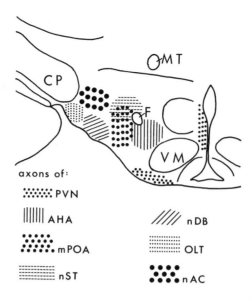

Figure 5.12 A cross-section through the medial forebrain bundle at the level of the ventro-medial hypothalamus (VM). As part of the tendency toward "laminar flow," a quasi-orderly pattern of descending projections, axons from more dorsal cell groups tend to run dorsally; lateral, laterally; medial, medially; and so forth (Pfaff & Conrad 1978).

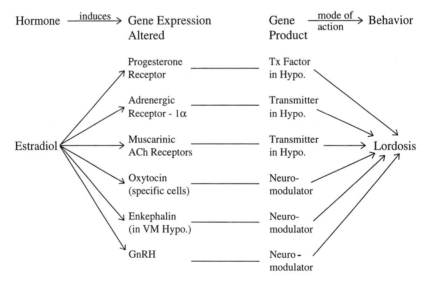

Figure 5.13 Hormone-gene-behavior "syllogisms." If estradiol administration induces gene expression in hypothalamic neurons and if the gene product in those neurons fosters re-productive behavior, it follows that these genomic effects represent mechanisms by which estradiol facilitates reproductive behavior. Different gene products have different modes of action in affecting behavior. For example, the progesterone receptor acts as a transcription factor (Tx factor) in hypothalamic neurons, whereas transmitter receptor induction favors neuro-transmitter action, and peptide induction favors neuromodulator action.

al. (1973). The neuroanatomy of these hormone-dependent neurons has been proved to be a stable story over almost 30 years. First published in early 1968, the pattern of a highly conserved neuroanatomical sex steroid receptor system accompanied by species-specific cell groups finds its extension, as the most recent example, in newts (Davis & Moore, 1996).

Throughout this neuroanatomical research, the original binding data have been confirmed and extended by immunocytochemical and in situ hybridization localization of gene products for hormone receptors (Lauber et al., 1990, 1991; Ricciardi & Blaustein, 1994; Romano et al., 1989; Simerly et al., 1996).

1. GENOMIC EFFECTS

Aside from the clear electrophysiological effects of estrogens (Bueno, 1976; Moss, 1997) and androgens (Pfaff & Pfaffmann, 1969) on preoptic or hypothalamic neurons, there are two physiologically crucial effects on gene expression. At least six neurochemical systems are turned on by estrogens, and their products, in turn, facilitate lordosis behavior (figure 5.13). In some cases, not only can a gene product that is a ligand be increased by estrogen, but also gene expression for its cognate receptor is heightened by estrogens, a "multiplicative" effect of the hormone (see chapter 10). Thus, we can say that the ER gene operates on lordosis by turning on at least six other genes important for the behavior (see also chapter 7).

Moreover, in turn, the behavioral necessity of the genes for the estrogen receptor and the progesterone receptor (both transcription factors) is proved by homologous recombination techniques in mice, which result in so-called gene knockouts (figure 5.14) for ERKO, "estrogen receptor gene knockout," and PRKO, "progesterone receptor gene knockout." To create gene knockouts, molecular geneticists synthesize nucleic acid sequences flanked by nucleotide bases identical to the gene in question. When this "Trojan Horse" nucleic acid sequence is administered artificially to embryonic stem cells, geneticists arrange, in a small percentage of cases, for the artificial sequence actually to be substituted for the normal gene. Then, when these cells are implanted in female mice, baby

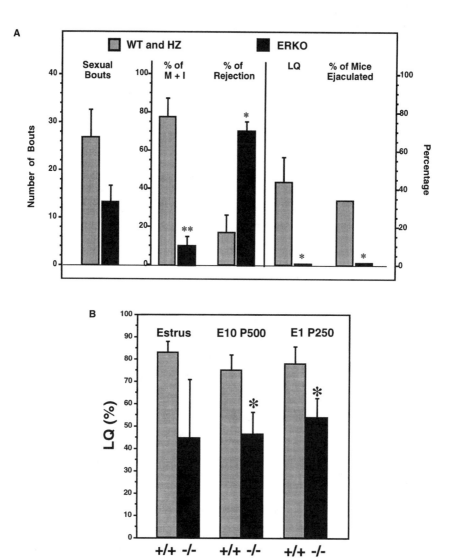

Figure 5.14 Comparisons of behaviors in estrogen receptor knockout (ERKO) ovari-ectomized female mice with wild-type mice (WT) and heterozygotes (HZ) (*top*), as well as progesterone receptor knockout (PRKO) ovariectomized female mice with wild-type females (*bottom*). (*Top*) Even under the influence of estradiol benzoate and progesterone (EB+P), ERKO female mice refused to show lordosis (LQ); thus, the stud males could not ejaculate. The ERKO females attracted less attention from the males (% Mounts + Intromissions) and rejected approaches by the males significantly more often. (From Ogawa et al., 1997, and unpublished data). (*Bottom*) Either before ovariectomy ("Estrus") or after ovariectomy treated with estradiol [E dose (in micrograms)] and progesterone [P dose (in micrograms)], PRKO females (−/−) could show a surprising amount of lordosis behavior (LQ), though less than wild-type females (+/+). In the original article regarding progesterone enhancement of female reproductive be-havior (Lydon et al., 1995) and in our hands, PRKO females do not show a significant facili-tation of estrogen-stimulated behavior by progesterone (P). (Ogawa et al., unpublished data.)

Table 5.2   Rapid, nongenomic actions of estrogens

Neuronal Communication	Nonneuronal Cells and Tissues
Membrane excitability of glutamate receptors	Binding to pituitary membranes
Changes in potency of mu-opioid receptors	Calcium influx on endometrial cells
Increase in intracellular calcium	Calcium influx in suspension of uterine cells
Neurotransmitter release and uptake	Calcium mobilization in granulosa and osteoblast cells
Increases in exo-endocytic pits and intramembrane particles	Effects on quality of maturing oocytes (fertilization and early postfertilization)
Immediate early gene products	Rapid prolactin release from pituitary tumor cells
Binding to neuronal membranes	Increase in membrane permeability: rapid increase in intracellular nucleoside activity
	Coronary tone in humans
	Spiking activity in pituitary
	Relaxation of smooth muscle

Source: From Moss et al., 1997.

mice are grown with the "Trojan Horse" knockout sequence in place of the normal gene in some cells and, eventually, in germ cells. Finally, such mice are mated to create an entire line of mice in which the relevant gene is deleted.

Estrogen receptor knockout female mice simply will not perform lordosis behavior (Ogawa et al., 1996b). Progesterone receptor knockout mice can perform lordosis of limited extent under certain circumstances (Ogawa et al., 1997), but the ability of progesterone to facilitate the estrogen effect on this behavior is much reduced (Lydon et al., 1995). Therefore, both in the requirements that for normal behavior the genes expressing the estrogen receptor and progesterone receptor must be actively transcribing *and* in the ability of hormones to influence gene expression for behaviorally important products in neurons, the relationships of individual genes to a specific behavior are proved (see chapter 7, figure 7.16).

Emphasizing these demonstrations of specific genomic contributions to a particular mammalian behavior does not mean that hormones cannot act in other ways. Estrogens can have rapid effects at the cell membrane (table 5.2; Moss, 1997). Progestins can act rapidly at the benzodiazepine portion of the GABA receptor (Baulieu, 1996; Freeman et al., 1993). Androgens can have rapid effects on preoptic neuron electrophysiology (Pfaff & Pfaffmann, 1969). These rapid membrane effects of steroids seem likely to complement, in unknown ways, the more time-consuming, genomic actions of sex hormones in the central nervous system.

D. SEX DIFFERENCES

Expression of the SRY gene on the Y chromosome eventually leads to the development of testes instead of ovaries. Resulting high levels of testosterone early in the life of the genetic male—the critical period for the rat brain being from birth until 5 days after birth—have at least two types of permanent effects on the developing male brain: loss of female-type behavioral and neuroendocrine functions (so-called defeminization) and increased male-typical functions (so-called masculinization). Surprisingly, for testosterone to have this effect, it had to be converted (aromatized) to estradiol. In fact, antisense DNA against the messenger RNA for the estrogen receptor delivered just before experimental neonatal testosterone treatment helped to preserve a female-typical behavior: lordosis (McCarthy et al., 1993). The sexually differentiating actions of both the estrogen receptor and the androgen receptor genes have been described in animals and human beings (figure 5.15). Mutations in the human androgen receptor gene or in the gene for steroid reductase type 2 lead to a failure of masculine secondary sexual characteristics, in turn leading to a female-type sexual identity (see also chapter 7).

The total array of estrogen receptor gene actions on sexual differentiation is more subtle and complex. On the one hand (as mentioned), local expression of the estrogen receptor messenger RNA, only in the hypothalamus and only during the neonatal period, is required for normal defeminization by neonatal

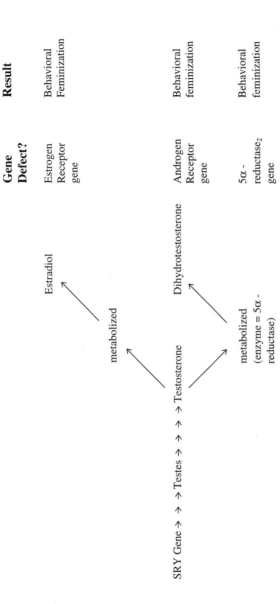

Figure 5.15   Several types of genetic deficiencies can interfere with the normal masculinization of behavior. Subsequent to the expression of the SRY gene in the genetic male, several steps permit development of the testes. As a result, testosterone is secreted. At least three genetic defects can prevent testosterone from leading to normal behavioral masculinization: an estrogen receptor gene knockout (Ogawa et al., 1997); mutations in the androgen receptor gene; and mutations in the type 2 5–α–reductase gene (Wilson et al., 1995.)

testosterone (McCarthy et al., 1993). On the other hand, estrogen receptor knockout female mice show a trend toward a masculine identity (Ogawa et al., 1996a,b) and, amazingly, estrogen receptor knockout male mice are partially feminized (Ogawa et al., 1997). Of course, with estrogen receptor gene knockouts, the failure of estrogen receptor gene expression is total throughout the body and during the entire life cycle. By putting all these data together, we can see that the impact of estrogen receptor gene expression on sexual differentiation depends (A) on on the gender of the animal in which the gene is expressed and (B) on exactly when and where in the body it is expressed (see figure 7.16 and chapter 7).

All these actions of genes during development will be classified as *indirect* effects of genes on subsequent adult behavior, as opposed to direct effects of the same gene (Ogawa et al., 1996b) on lordosis behavior in adulthood (see chapter 7).

The resulting behavioral effects of the classical androgen receptor gene and estrogen receptor gene during normal development in animals and in human beings submit to a broad summary. Behaviors closely associated with reproduction are impressively different between males and females in humans and other animals, but behaviors not associated with reproduction, including a variety of cognitive functions, are by and large similar between males and females. For example, in rats, copulatory behaviors and neuroendocrine controls over the pituitary are beautifully physiologically coordinated and differ strikingly between males and females (see figure 5.4). Moreover, those communications and courtship behaviors that bring male and female together in a hormonally dependent fashion—the communication and courtship sequences depending on androgens in the male and estrogens in the female—likewise are sexually differentiated (Floody & Pfaff, 1977; Pfaff et al., 1972). Severe aggression is more typical in males, but compared to these huge, reliable behavioral differences in lower animals, the evidence in humans for sex differences in higher cognitive or cultural capacities is of a weak statistical sort.

Throughout the story of sexual differentiation, the connections of gene expression to behavior have been clear. Even less direct effects of gene expression during development, connected with the migration of gonadotropin-releasing hormone neurons from the nose to the brain, have been adduced in the genesis of Kallmann's syndrome, in which human males lack libido (see chapters 7 and 10).

E. SUMMARY

Hormones can determine behavior powerfully through actions that use specific chemical steps in specific parts of the brain. Behaviors influenced in this way include both particular instinctive responses and broader motivational states. Some of these behaviors show marked sex differences, the mechanisms of which have been explored. The effects of gene expression on sexually differentiated behaviors are clear. However, we also show that the effect of a given gene on a given behavior can depend on the gender in which that gene is expressed and on exactly where and when during development it is expressed (see chapter 7).

How can hormones act in such a manner as to influence an individual mammalian molar behavior? The answer requires analysis of the neural circuitry involved.

6

Neural Explanation of Hormone-Controlled Drive

The system is the solution.

—Recent TV ad

Neurobiologists have come a long way toward explaining the cellular bases of sensation and perception as would underlie the laws of psychophysics. Perhaps the most striking progress has been made in the visual system, where the fundamental advances led by David Hubel and Torsten Wiesel brought us all the way from the retinal surface through several layers of processing in the cerebral cortex. Likewise, considering motor responses, the synaptic physiology and reflex motor control elucidated by Sir John Eccles and his many colleagues laid open the subject in a way that would have pleased his former mentor, Sir Charles Sherrington. But what about unraveling the mechanisms that form the underpinning for an entire behavioral system, a molar behavioral response of a mammal?

For a neurobiologist to be successful, a behavior must be selected carefully, one simple enough actually to be explainable. Hormone-driven female-typical reproductive behaviors serve as a good choice for several reasons. First, the very fact that such hormones as estradiol and progesterone drive these behaviors has helped because we were able to find out precisely where in the central nervous system such steroid hormones acted. Then all the tools of cellular and molecular endocrinology could be brought into play. Second, the simplicity of the behavior itself has been a tremendous aid. Lordosis behavior, typical of female quadrupeds, simply is a standing response coupled with a vertebral dorsiflexion. This behavior requires that the female stop other activities, especially locomotion, and adopt a rigid enough, bilaterally symmetrical posture, to allow the male to mount and to support his weight. Then, arching the back permits fertilization by the male. This behavior occurs only with the proper schedule of priming with estrogens followed by amplification with progesterone. The behavior is a hormone-sensitive response to a specific cutaneous stimulus, the first skin contact from the male; if the female will not perform this response because of insufficient estradiol or progesterone, the male's mounts will be to no avail. Third, the behavior is biologically crucial. Without lordosis, fertilization will not occur. Thus, through this behavior, the female's hormonal state determines her own biological investment in reproduction for the next few days or weeks.

We figured out the neural circuitry for this behavior (1) by starting with the hormone effects and working out from the hypothalamus (2) by starting with the simple tactile stimuli that triggered the behavior and working our way up the neuraxis, and (3) by working backward from the simple motor behavioral response into the motor control pathways.

A. A NEURAL CIRCUIT FOR A MAMMALIAN MATING BEHAVIOR

The neural circuit for female rat lordosis behavior (figure 6.1) has been presented in detail (Pfaff, 1980; Pfaff et al., 1994). As the evidence establishing this circuit has been published *in extenso,* only a few of the main points are illustrated here. *It is important to note that in explaining the hormone effect on this mating behavior, we are at the same time explaining a simple form of sexual motivation.*

Lordosis is triggered by cutaneous stimulation on the flanks of female rats followed by pressure on the posterior rump, tail base, and perineum. This pressure is applied by the male rat during natural mating behavior, is necessary for lordosis to occur, and is sufficient for lordosis behavior. Such cutaneous stimulation, applied by the male rat and leading to lordosis, can cause a barrage of action potentials from most of the cutaneous mechanoreceptive unit types in the dorsal root ganglia. However, among all primary sensory neurons, only pressure units and type I units (figure 6.2) gave sustained responses to a lordosis-triggering type of cutaneous pressure stimulation. These types of sensory units had requirements that most closely fit the pattern of stimulus requirements for lordosis behavior as a whole. To evoke lordosis behavior, summation across pressure units certainly occurs, and summation with other unit types also may be involved. If any single chain of events has the central role in the behavior, however, it is that pressure on the crucial skin areas deforms a special class of cutaneous receptors named *Ruffini endings,* thereby activating pressure units. Determining precise stimulus requirements for the lordosis circuit to function was important, because the specificity of the behavioral result depends not only on hormone action and gene transcription but on the exact nature of the sensory input.

Behaviorally important sensory information triggers massive discharges in neurons deep in the rat dorsal horn of the spinal cord. However, local spinal circuits by themselves are not sufficient for lordosis behavior. Instead, lordosis behavior requires a long circuit comprising ascending sensory information and descending neuronal facilitation from supraspinal nerve cell groups. The critical ascending and descending pathways run in the anterolateral columns of the spinal cord. The behaviorally important targets of the ascending fibers in lordosis behavior circuitry are in the medullary reticular formation and the lateral vestibular nucleus (see figure 6.1). Some fibers also make it to the midbrain central gray. Ascending sensory terminations in the brainstem do not immediately control descending neurons in a simple and direct manner; the subsequent descending facilitation of lordosis behavior by brainstem neurons appears not simply to be the result of a spinal-brainstem-spinal reflex but rather a tonic nature that reflects, in part, durable estrogenic influences originating in the hypothalamus.

At the top of the circuitry that facilitates lordosis behavior are the nerve cells in and immediately surrounding the ventromedial nucleus of the hypothalamus. Lesions or pharmacological blockage of these cells leads to a loss of

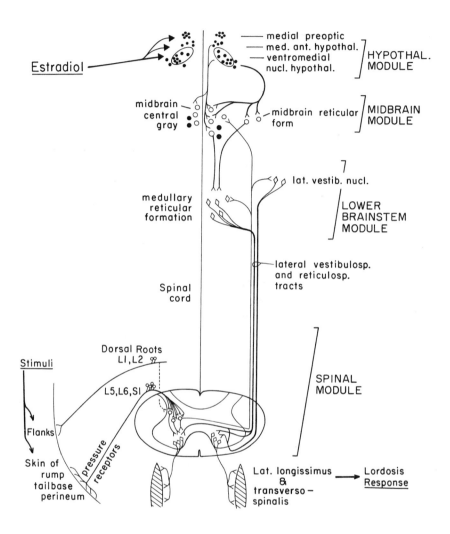

Estradiol

medial preoptic
med. ant. hypothal.
ventromedial
nucl. hypothal.
HYPOTHAL.
MODULE

midbrain
central
gray

midbrain reticular
form
MIDBRAIN
MODULE

lat. vestib. nucl.

medullary
reticular
formation
LOWER
BRAINSTEM
MODULE

lateral vestibulosp.
and reticulosp.
tracts

Spinal
cord

Stimuli

Dorsal Roots
LI, L2

L5, L6, SI

SPINAL
MODULE

Flanks

Skin of
rump
tailbase
perineum

pressure
receptors

Lat. longissimus
&
transverso-
spinalis

Lordosis
Response

lordosis behavior. Electrical stimulation of these cells leads to lordosis facilitation. No other lesion or electrical stimulation sites in the forebrain can account for the facilitation of lordosis behavior by forebrain tissue. Therefore, among all telencephalic and diencephalic sites, the main source of lordosis behavior facilitation must be ventromedial hypothalamic neurons.

The organization of axons descending from the hypothalamus has begun to be sorted out. Those axons related to lordosis behavior descend from the ventromedial hypothalamus either through a medial periventricular trajectory or through a lateral sweeping trajectory back to the midbrain reticular formation

Figure 6.1 Sketch of the basic neural circuit for producing the primary female reproductive behavior, lordosis. (From Pfaff et al., 1994.) This was the first completed neural circuit for a vertebrate behavior. Cutaneous stimuli triggering pressure receptors on the flanks and then the hindquarters of the female rat evoke action potentials entering the spinal cord over dorsal roots L1, L2, L5, L6, and S1. Although the responses by neurons in appropriate parts of the dorsal horn are prompt and impressive, spinal tissue by itself cannot mediate lordosis behavior. The obligatory ascending fibers in the supraspinal loop travel to the brainstem in the anterolateral columns, terminating in considerable numbers in the medullary reticular formation and dorsocaudal lateral vestibular nucleus and, in less quantity, in the midbrain (the peripenduncular region and the midbrain central gray). The main job of the hypothalamic module in this circuit is to add estrogen and progestin dependence. Operating through estrogen receptors expressed in ventromedial hypothalamic neurons, estradiol induces expression of the gene for the progesterone receptor, and circulating progesterone binds to that receptor. Their combined genomic and electrophysiological effects send an enabling signal back to the midbrain central gray over both axons that follow a sweeping lateral route and a smaller number of axons that follow a periventricular route. Then, neurons in the dorsal lateral portion of the midbrain central gray, combined with a smaller number of neurons in the nearby mesencephalic reticular formation, send a descending signal that facilitates medullary reticulospinal neurons. Reticulospinal signals synergize with lateral vestibulospinal discharges (e.g., see figure 6.3) to facilitate activity in the lumbar motor neurons that lie on the medial side of the ventral horn and are responsible for controlling the deep back muscles—the lateral longisimus and transversospinalis. On reception of adequate sensory input, these motor neurons allow muscle contraction that changes the posture of the back to "concave up," which drives lordosis behavior and thus permits fertilization. Modules in this circuit match embryological divisions of the developing mammalian central nervous system (see figure 6.8). Three of these modules are shown in slightly greater detail, in cross-section, in figure 6.6.

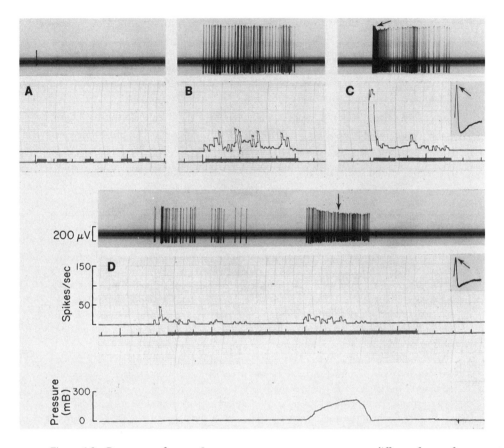

Figure 6.2 Responses of a type I pressure-receptor sensory neuron to different forms of stimulation. Each time division denotes 1 second. (*A*) Air puffs, (*B*) Brushing, (*C*) Von Frey-hair, (*D*) Pressure. A response was evoked by mere contact with the pressure-sensitive receptive field on the skin and then by the small amount of pressure at the very beginning of pressure application. Despite reductions in spike amplitude during responses, the shape of the action potential remained the same, as shown by the inserts in panels *C* and *D* (taken from the spike trains, as indicated by arrows). (From Kow & Pfaff, 1979.)

and periaqueductal gray. Those axons descending through a lateral sweeping trajectory make a larger quantitative contribution to lordosis. Neurons in the central gray send axons descending into the medullary reticular formation. The descending central gray signal activates medullary reticulospinal neurons as they synergize with lateral vestibulospinal neurons to control the deep back muscles that execute lordosis (Cottingham et al., 1987, 1988; figure 6.3).

This midbrain central gray module is crucial. Electrical stimulation of the midbrain central gray will facilitate lordosis, whereas central gray lesions disrupt it. The physiology of central gray neurons also allows us to understand how a strong somatosensory stimulus from the male, which ordinarily would be treated as noxious, can lead to a reproductive behavior. The same subregions of the central gray of the midbrain that are important for lordosis behavior (when activated) will lead to a decrease in pain (Bodnar et al., 1998). They cause stimulus-dependent analgesia. Thus, we can see how their activation by hormonally dependent inputs from the hypothalamus and by perineal stimuli from the male actually permits the lordosis response to occur.

The synergizing input from the lateral vestibular nucleus also is important, as lesions there will reduce lordosis in proportion to the number of vestibulospinal cells destroyed, and electrical stimulation of the lateral vestibular nucleus will facilitate lordosis (figure 6.4). The lateral vestibulospinal tract from the lateral vestibular nucleus and the lateral reticulospinal tract from the medullary reticular formation are the descending pathways that facilitate lordosis. They enhance the throughput from behaviorally adequate sensory stimulation to the deep back muscle motor neurons (figure 6.5; Cohen et al., 1987). These descending systems themselves and the muscle groups that execute lordosis behavior have physiological properties absolutely congruent with the requirements of lordosis behavior as a whole (tables 6.1 and 6.2; Knobil & Neill, 1994).

The deep back muscles (named *lateral longissimus* and *transversospinalis*) are attached dorsally to the spinal column so that when they contract, the spinal column will be bent "concave up." Thus, these muscles are positioned perfectly to execute the vertebral dorsiflexion of lordosis and so are responsible for the

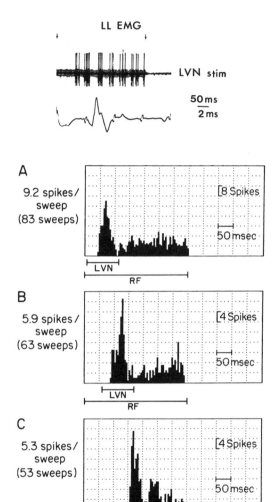

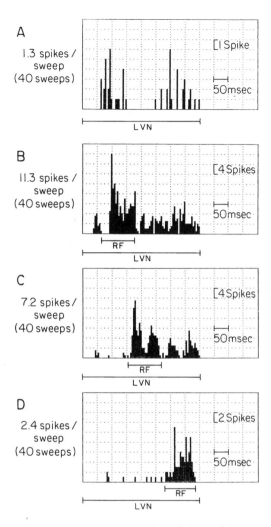

Figure 6.3 Descending excitation in the lateral vestibulospinal [originating in the lateral vestibular nucleus (LVN)] synergizes with medullary reticulospinal descending influences [originating in the medullary reticular formation (RF)] to excite motoneurons governing the deep back muscle lateral longisimus (LL), which is active in lordosis behavior. (From Cottingham et al., 1988.) (*Opposite, top*) Action potentials in the deep back muscle (LL). An electromyographic excitation caused by lateral vestibular nucleus stimulation (LVN). Bottom trace is a time-expanded record of one spike to show its unitary nature. (*Opposite, bottom*) Superimposition of LVN stimulation synergizes with a background of medullary RF stimulation to enhance deep back-muscle firing. (*Above*) The same type of experiment as on p. 84 but reversed. That is, superimposition of medullary RF stimulation synergizes with a background of LVN stimulation to enhance firing of the deep back muscle lateral longisimus, active in lordosis behavior.

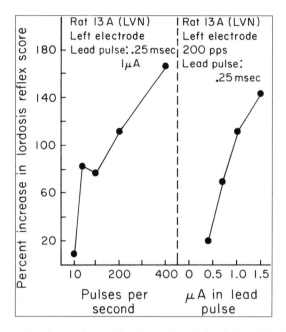

Figure 6.4   Lordosis reflex amplitude following unilateral stimulation of the lateral vestibular nucleus (LVN). (*Left*) All stimulation parameters except pulse frequency were kept constant in this series of tests. (*Right*) All stimulation parameters except amperage in the leading, cathodal pulse were kept constant in this series of tests. (From Modianos & Pfaff, 1977.)

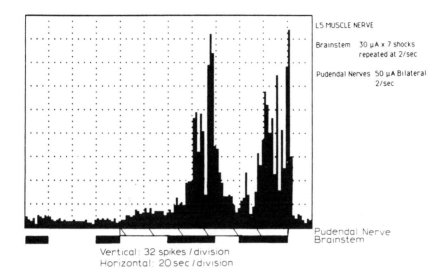

Vertical: 32 spikes / division
Horizontal: 20 sec / division

Figure 6.5 Quantitative summary of recordings from a deep back–muscle nerve (lateral longissimus), illustrating the synergistic effect of sensory input (pudendal nerve stimulation) and descending facilitation from the brainstem medullary reticular formation. That is, sensory stimulation by itself had little effect, and brainstem stimulation by itself had no effect. But, brainstem stimulation markedly potentiated the ability of sensory input from the pudendal nerve to evoke electrical activity in deep back–muscle motor neurons. (From Cohen et al., 1987.)

Table 6.1   Congruence of spinal neuronal and back muscle properties with behavioral requirements

---

Dynamic properties:

• Fast-twitch muscle (lateral longissimus) with few muscle spindles

   Weak monosynaptic reflex from Ia afferents

   Behavior does not have variable load, or "target"; is ballistic

• Fast axial muscles have large twitch tensions

   Maximum force needed to support weight of male

Spatial properties:

• Bilateral motoneuronal outputs to back muscles synergize to produce greater upward force

   Cutaneous stimuli and behavioral responses are bilaterally symmetrical

• Synaptic inputs from different spinal segments increase the output of axial motoneuron pool

   Cutaneous stimuli derive from multiple dermatomes, and dorsiflexion response extends across spinal segments

---

Source: From Pfaff et al., 1994, p. 163.

rump elevation, the most crucial component of lordosis behavior that allows fertilization by the male. These muscles are connected so as to be anatomically competent to execute the lordosis response, and they are electrically active during the initiation of lordosis behavior. Bilateral electrical stimulation of the lateral longissimus or transversospinalis muscles produces vertebral dorsiflexion. Ablation of these muscles reduces lordosis strength.

The motor neurons for these muscles lie on the medial and ventral side of the ventral horn. They can be found at spinal levels receiving dorsal roots from thoracic level 12 through sacral level 1 (i.e., just anterior to, in, and just posterior to the lumbar enlargement).

Thus, we have a brief summary of lordosis behavior circuitry from sensory input, through brainstem and hypothalamic control, to motor output. This circuitry was the first for any molar mammalian behavior and so proved the possibility of unraveling mechanisms for a mammalian behavior.

Table 6.2   Congruence of descending motor control system properties with behavioral requirements

---

- Reticulospinal and lateral vestibulospinal stimulation activates deep back–muscle EMG.

  RST and LVST control medial motoneurons and proximal muscles, in part through monosynaptic connections.

  Lesions of RS or LVN neurons, or severing their axons, decreases lordosis behavior; stimulating LVN increases it.

- Reticulospinal stimulation facilitates axial motoneuron response to pudendal nerve input.

  Descending hormone-modulated impulses and cutaneous stimuli control lordotic dorsiflexion.

- RST and LVST effects on back-muscle EMG increase with continued stimulation.

  Hormone-dependent hypothalamic output yields tonic input to RST.

- RST and LVST effects on spinal cord are bilateral

  Behavioral response is bilaterally symmetrical

- RST and LVST axons terminate at several spinal levels.

  Lordotic dorsiflexion response extends across spinal segments.

EMG, electromyography; RST, reticulospinal tract; LVST, lateral vestibulospinal tract; RS, reticulospinal; LVN, lateral vertibular nucleus.
Source: From Pfaff et al., 1994, p. 175.

1. MODULES IN THE CIRCUIT

Some of the separate modules in the lordosis behavior circuit are illustrated (figure 6.6; Knobil & Neill, 1994). Each module has its job. The *spinal cord module* obviously receives the major impact of somatosensory input, filters that input in each spinal cord segment, receives the descending facilitatory signals, and generates the motor neuronal output. Intersegmental facilitations we have described help to account for the overall vertebral dorsiflexion that characterizes the behavior.

The *lower brainstem module* integrates postural adaptations across spinal cord segments. The animal could not maintain a standing posture without adequate

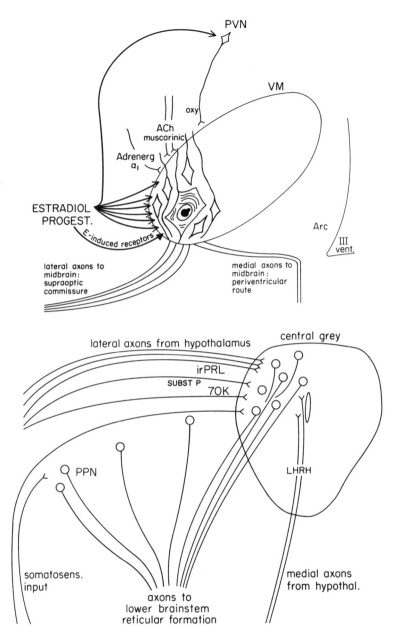

Figure 6.6 Four of the modules drawn schematically in cross-section, at different levels of the lordosis behavior circuitry (summarized in figure 6.1). (From Pfaff et al., 1994.) In the *hypothalamic module* (*above, top*), estradiol acting through the product of the estrogen receptor gene induces expression of the gene for the progesterone receptor. Estradiol and progesterone enhance sensitivity to α1 adrenergic agonists, to cholinergic muscarinic agonists, and to oxytocin (pictured) as well as to gonadotropin-releasing hormone (GnRH) and the opioid peptide enkephalin (not pictured). Axons descending from the ventromedial hypothalamic

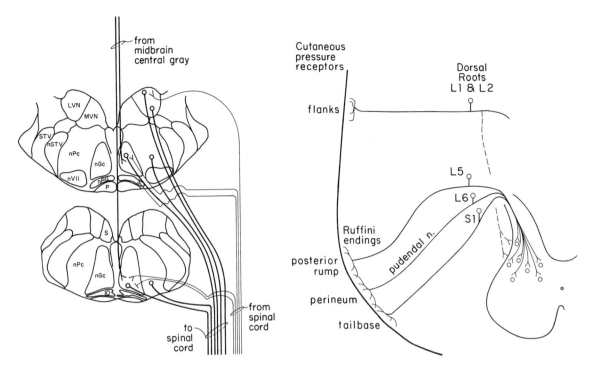

nucleus (VM) take either a lateral, sweeping route through the supraoptic commissure to the midbrain module or a medial periventricular route. In the *midbrain module,* the dorsolateral portion of the midbrain central gray receives a large excitatory input from the ventromedial hypothalamus, both from a sweeping lateral trajectory and from a medial periventricular route. Among other substances, these axons carry prolactin substance P, an estrogen-induced protein the molecular weight of which is approximately 70,000 (HIP 70; Mobbs et al., 1988, 1990). Also, small numbers of GnRH-containing (GnRH, LHRH) axons ascend into the medial portion of the midbrain central gray, following a periventricular route. Finally, at the midbrain level, the peripeduncular nucleus (PPN) and the midbrain central gray receive a significant somatosensory input due to signals from the mating partner. Note, however, that this input is not as quantitatively strong as that received by the lower brainstem module, which in turn is not as strong as the spinal cord module. Axons from the dorsal lateral central gray and the peripeduncular region descend to the hindbrain module, where they synapse in the reticular formation, which in turn will synergize with lateral vestibulospinal mechanisms. In the *hindbrain (lower brainstem) module (above, left),* neurons in both the medullary reticular formation and in the dorsocaudal portion of the lateral vestibular nucleus (LVN) receive heavy somatosensory inputs from the spinal cord, which ascended through the anterolateral columns. The portion of the reticular formation called *nucleus gigantocellularis* (nGc) also receives an enabling input from the midbrain central gray. Together, axons from the medullary reticular formation and the lateral vestibulospinal nucleus (LVN) descend through the anterolateral columns of the spinal cord to facilitate lordosis behavior. In the *spinal cord module (above, right),* following cutaneous pressure bilaterally on the flanks (entering the spinal cord over dorsal roots L1 and L2), pressure on Ruffini endings in the skin of the posterior rump, perineum, and tail base, which leads to action potentials entering the spinal cord over L5, L6, and S1, excite second-order neurons deep in the ipsilateral dorsal horn.

input from vestibular organs (which sense the head's position and movement) and proprioceptors (which sense skeletal and muscle movement) up and down the length of the body. Because the spinal cord is organized primarily segment by segment, neuronal groups above the spinal cord are required to achieve this integration.

The *midbrain module* serves as the receiving zone for hypothalamic and preoptic peptides and proteins of neuroendocrine import. It translates signals coming from the hypothalamus, which have a very slow time course typical of neuroendocrine mechanisms, into faster-changing electrophysiological signals typical of the rest of the nervous system. Hierarchically, central gray neurons facilitate reticulospinal cells in the lower brainstem module.

The *hypothalamic module* adds the primary endocrine control component to this behavioral mechanism. Steroid hormone binding and the genomic effects (see chapter 7) of estrogens and progestins, resulting in electrical activation, account for the strong steroid hormone dependence of the neural circuit and lordosis behavior as a whole.

Up through the hypothalamic module, the nerve cells responsible for actually producing the behavior have been accounted for. The major role of cell groups in the *forebrain module* is to inhibit the behavior, with the exception of certain pheromonal inputs (see later).

A series of articles from the laboratory of Yasuo Sakuma in Tokyo and work from Lee-Ming Kow quoted here have supported elegantly the notion that with respect both to lordosis and to foregoing courtship behaviors, estrogen increases excitability of specific cell groups within the medial hypothalamus and preoptic area (POA), respectively (figure 6.7). That is, estrogen increases reproductive drive in two ways: First, in preoptic neurons, which foster locomotion (Smith, 1997), approach, and courtship behaviors. Then, estrogen turns on a subset of ventromedial hypothalamic neurons that have very low initial spontaneous activity (Bueno & Pfaff, 1976) and that also respond to glucose (signaling adequate food supply), norepinephrine (signaling adequate arousal), and oxytocin. Because POA neuronal physiology frequently opposes hypothalamic effects and because female rats always require the sudden cessation of rapid (POA-dependent) locomotion to initiate (ventromedial hypothalamus–dependent) lordosis, we offer the concept that the physiological opposition between the two mechanisms enforces a sequential performance of the two behaviors: courtship and (only then) lordosis.

We have noticed that modules in the lordosis behavior circuit defined by neuroanatomical and electrophysiological evidence reflect divisions apparent during embryological development (figure 6.8; Knobil & Neill, 1994). The consonance of the neural circuit for this behavior with embryologically important segments of the neuraxis increased even more our confidence that we had gotten the circuit "right."

2. DESCENDING SYSTEMS SYNERGIZE TO PRODUCE A TAUT POSTURAL BACKGROUND ON WHICH SPECIFIC CUTANEOUS STIMULI ARE IMPOSED

One could suppose that a simple mating behavior would be organized by targeted stimuli ascending to behaviorally dedicated control circuits in the midbrain and forebrain, thus to trigger behaviorally dedicated descending systems. That is not the way things work. Instead, massive descending systems crucial for a variety of postural adaptations synergize to produce an organism with extremely tense posture, receptive in the extreme to behaviorally adequate cutaneous stimuli.

Reticulospinal systems (projecting from the medullary reticular formation to the spinal cord) and vestibulospinal systems [projecting from the lateral vestibular nucleus (LVN) to the spinal cord] cooperate to produce the postural background against which lordosis behavior can be evoked. Electromyographic (EMG) activity evoked in axial muscles by LVN stimulation can be facilitated by concurrent stimulation of nucleus gigantocellularis of the reticular formation (Cottingham et al., 1988). Indeed, behaviorally facilitatory sites in nucleus gigantocellularis are precisely those that at higher currents could themselves activate axial motor units. Facilitation of the response to vestibulospinal stimulation by reticular stimulation is manifested both as an increased number of EMG units

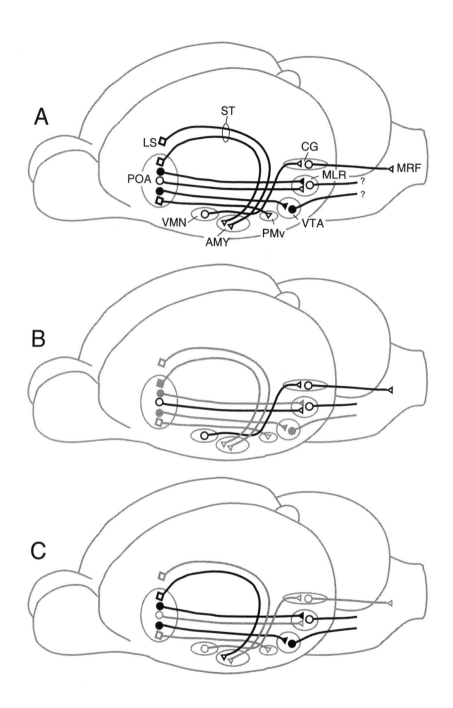

firing in response to a given LVN stimulus intensity and as a decrease in threshold for vestibulospinal activation of axial EMG units.

The reticular formation effects themselves are facilitated by the midbrain central gray. The effect of midbrain central gray stimulation was to lower the threshold for reticular formation–evoked EMG activity, to decrease the latency of the axial muscle response with respect to the onset of the reticular formation train, and to increase the number of EMG units to respond (Appelberg et al., 1967; Carlson,1978; Cottingham, 1986; Cottingham et al.,1987).

Figure 6.7 Beyond the basic neural circuit demonstrated to *facilitate* lordosis behavior, certain cell groups in the forebrain (telencephalic module) can *inhibit* lordosis behavior. The electrophysiological experiments of Sakuma have revealed how such cell groups as the preoptic area (POA), amygdala (AMY), and lateral septum (LS) communicate with hypothalamus and midbrain to inhibit female reproductive behavior, especially in the male rat. (*A*) "Hardwiring" of the circuitry discovered in Sakuma's work. The flow of electrical impulses dominant in the male rat (Sakuma, 1984; Sakuma & Pfaff, 1981), with some modulation by androgenic hormones in the male (Suga & Sakuma, 1994). Filled circles denote nerve cell bodies that send off *inhibitory* synapses. Open circles denote neurons with *excitatory* synaptic outputs. For the neurons shown by open diamonds, synaptic characteristics are not yet known. In the male, preoptic neurons inhibit midbrain cell groups such as the midbrain locomotor region (MLR) and the ventral tegmental area (VTA), both of which appear (Sakamoto et al., 1993) to send descending axons to the medullary reticular formation (MRF). There, they facilitate proceptive behaviors that lead to lordosis. (*B*) In the estrogen-treated female rat, neuronal impulse flow from the ventromedial nucleus of the hypothalamus (VMN) through the midbrain to the medullary reticular formation (MRF) is augmented greatly and uses an important excitatory synaptic link in the midbrain central gray (CG) (Akaishi & Sakuma, 1986; Sakuma, 1984; Sakuma & Akaishi, 1987; Sakuma & Pfaff, 1980a,b, 1981, 1982; Sakuma & Tada, 1984). Importantly, estrogen facilitates the excitatory POA effects on the midbrain locomotor region (MLR), for stimulating courtship behaviors while it supresses the inhibitory effects (Sakuma, 1994; Takeo & Sakuma, 1995). POA outputs to the amygdala (AMY) and the VTA also are suppressed (Hasegawa & Sakuma, 1993; Takeo & Sakuma, 1995). (*C*) In the female rat lacking estrogen, *inhibitory* outputs prevail from the POA to the MLR (Sakuma, 1994) and to the VTA (Hasegawa & Sakuma, 1993). In contrast, POA projections to the ventral premammillary nucleus (Nakano et al., 1997) as well as septal projections to the AMY (Yoshida et al., 1994) are not sensitive to estrogen. In summary, estrogens facilitate preoptic outputs that will foster courtship or sex behaviors in the female, and they inhibit preoptic outputs that would block those behaviors.

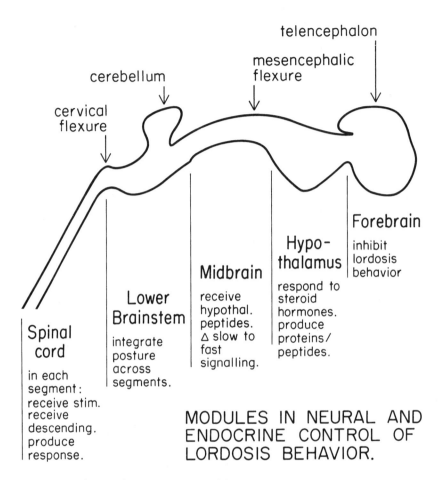

cervical flexure

cerebellum

mesencephalic flexure

telencephalon

Forebrain
inhibit lordosis behavior

Hypo-thalamus
respond to steroid hormones. produce proteins/peptides.

Midbrain
receive hypothal. peptides. Δ slow to fast signalling.

Lower Brainstem
integrate posture across segments.

Spinal cord
in each segment: receive stim. receive descending. produce response.

MODULES IN NEURAL AND ENDOCRINE CONTROL OF LORDOSIS BEHAVIOR.

Figure 6.8   The central nervous system modules in the lordosis behavior circuitry as determined (Pfaff, 1980; Pfaff et al., 1994) precisely match the major neuraxis divisions, or segments, of the embryonic nervous system (sketched in simplified form). Each module has a major functional role in the regulation of female reproductive behavior. (From Pfaff et al., 1994.)

Thus, the specificity in the control of lordosis behavior does not lie solely in the choice of particular vestibulospinal or reticulospinal axons, nor does it lie in their individual properties. The very anatomical and physiological properties that render these systems ideal for the control of lordosis behavior (see tables 6.1 and 6.2) show us that their broad distribution across spinal levels on both sides of the spinal cord would not permit them to pick out one behavior by themselves for facilitation. Instead, the postural background impressively established by these two descending systems allows for a *codetermination* of lordosis behavior by the confluence of hormonal actions in the hypothalamus and the adequate sensory stimulus from the mounting male.

A series of properties of lordosis behavior circuitry show us splendidly how the organization of a neural system can be economical in its use of neurally integrative features and in its adaptation of behavior to the environment. First is the obvious economy in the use of ascending sensory information. The distribution of cutaneous information for triggering lordosis behavior is limited and selective, operating on the need-to-know principle. At several points in the neural circuit for lordosis behavior, obviously not all sensory information is transferred from one module to the next (reviewed in Pfaff et al., 1994). Correspondingly, the increasing size of receptive fields along the lordosis behavior circuit provides for the convergence of information necessary for the adequate summation of stimuli in the determination of the behavior (see later).

Summation

A punctate stimulus on a square micrometer of skin rarely is the sole determinant of a molar behavior. Instead, stimuli must be summated across receptor fields to achieve a given behavior. The sensory controls that have been reported for lordosis behavior (Pfaff, 1980) show that the convergence of receptive fields for different locations on the skin within lordosis sensory pathways in fact achieves enough stimulus summation to trigger lordosis behavior. Both summation across skin area and summation across modalities of cutaneous sensitivity provide the behavior-triggering power that lordosis as a molar, complete behavior actually requires.

Interactions

Further, within lordosis circuitry mechanisms, at least three different kinds of interactions provide for the proper management of the behavior. First, *stimulus-stimulus interactions* within and between sensory modalities arrange for the biologically appropriate occurrence of the behavior. Within modality, summation (as described) can occur. Between modalities, the addition of olfactory stimuli from the male, for example, to somatosensory stimuli from the male's mounting behavior can provide for a longer and stronger lordosis. Second, *hormone-stimulus interactions* occur most obviously when the application of estrogens and progestins increases the likelihood that a given set of stimuli will lead to a greater behavioral response (Kow et al., 1979; Pfaff et al., 1977). Third, *hormone-hormone interactions* are illustrated clearly when estrogen leads to increased gene expression for the progesterone receptor, in turn to facilitate the behaviorally important actions of progesterone (see chapter 7). Likewise, the interactions of thyroid hormonal systems with estrogen-responsive systems increase the possibility that disruptive environmental stimuli not consistent with reproduction will interfere with estrogen-dependent neuroendocrine mechanisms.

Ethological Concepts

As a side point, the neural circuitry for these natural mammalian behavior patterns and the hormone effects on them explain some of the long-held, classic concepts of ethology as formulated during the epoch-making animal behavior studies of Lorenz (1970) and Tinbergen (1951). Matching their types of behavioral concepts with our physiological explanations is surprisingly simple. For example, the *ethological concept of a sign stimulus* is that a selected set of stimulus energies is required to evoke a selected behavioral response (Tinbergen, 1951). "Sign stimuli," though sometimes specified along a single physical scale, more frequently can act through more than one modality (Hinde, 1966). They can be thought of as switching on and directing motivated behaviors (Gould, 1982). A releasing mechanism, composed essentially of a stimulus-filtering process, provides the key to the relevant motor mechanism. This is seen easily in the physiology of lordosis behavior: Stimuli for evoking lordosis behavior are restricted not only as to their modality but also according to a specific cutaneous input from certain places on the skin of the female rat. In turn, electrophysiological recordings of the relevant inputs from primary sensory neurons and from interneurons in the spinal cord, along with circuitry analyses of how lordosis behavioral responses occur, provide the physiological explanation of how such sign stimuli work (Pfaff, 1980).

Likewise, the concept of a *fixed action pattern* is a natural behavioral response that is a movement of constant form. The concept simply derives from the main ethological methods for the description and classification of behavior (Hinde, 1966, p. 11). Its definition includes the idea that well-coordinated subunits of the behavior have a fixed relation to each other, with each subunit having innate, stereotyped characteristics (Gould, 1982, p. 37, p. 163–164). The detailed description of lordosis behavior based on high-speed film and x-ray analyses (chapter 1 in Pfaff, 1980) and on the anatomical and physiological studies of the muscular basis for lordosis response execution transparently fits the definition of a fixed action pattern.

Finally, Lorenz's simplest model (Gould, 1982, illustration on p. 186) for the *motivation of instinctive behavioral responses* can be used as a description of the most elementary hormonal effects on rodent mating behavior. Operationally, from a black-box point of view, estrogen provides Lorenz's motivational "hydraulic pressure" for the lordosis behavior response to occur. More generally, in modern ethology, a motivational effect would be used to explain a change in responsiveness to a constant external stimulus (Hinde, 1966). Neurochemical studies (summarized in Pfaff et al., 1994) and genetic studies (summarized partially in chapter 7) provide the mechanisms for such a motivational influence.

Thus, the phenomena and mechanisms for female reproductive behavior in rodents not only are consistent with some of the key concepts in ethology;

their neural and molecular analysis provides physiological explanations for etho-logical concepts in an interesting context.

3. Principle: Determination of a Behavior

The principle established by this brief mechanistic description and the more complete set of references previously published (Pfaff, 1980; Pfaff et al., 1994) is as follows. A particular molar mammalian behavior is determined by a speci-fic neural circuit stretching from lumbar spinal cord stimulus input up to the midbrain. In the midbrain, circuit excitability is elevated by descending influ-ences from hormone-dependent neurons in the hypothalamus, thus to facilitate a motor control system that descends back to the lumbar spinal cord. In the lumbar cord, deep back-muscle motoneurons execute lordosis behavior. This specific neural system determining a particular mammalian behavior provides for the intersection of hormonal influences and stimulus triggers acting on the behavior.

B. Orchestration of External and Internal Influences on Biologically Appropriate Reproduction, Using the Circuit

The preceding section shows how hormones and environment can interact to produce a particular behavior. However, the only aspect of the environment considered was the sensory input from the male, a brief and specific input. Now we open this subject more broadly, considering interactions of the female with her environment over a longer period of time before sex behavior (sections B1 and B2). Also, we consider a much wider range of environmental factors (sec-tions C1 and C2). The confluence of environmental thinking (from a zoo-logical point of view) with molecular biological technique and our knowledge of lordosis behavior circuitry allows for several examples of how the central nervous system integrates hormonal and environmental input to determine be-havior in a biologically adaptive fashion.

1. Female-Male Communications Forming a "Hormone-Dependent Behavioral Funnel"

Over long time courses before the female and male actually meet and during the short time course of their mating encounters, hormone-dependent responses in the female tend to encourage the next hormone response by the male, and vice versa. For example, under the influence of estrogens, females increase their locomotion and, in doing so, spread estrous odors (Pfaff et al., 1972, 1980). In turn, male rats under the influence of their androgens guide themselves up the olfactory gradient when they smell the female estrous odor until they contact the female rat, and so forth (figure 6.9).

Likewise, with female hamsters, hormone-dependent responses to olfactory stimuli and ultrasound stimuli foster the more intense behavioral interactions of female and male hamsters, which will lead to lordosis behavior. In a variety of animals, a virtual symphony of hormone-dependent courtship behaviors fosters later reproductive behaviors (figure 6.10; Floody & Pfaff, 1977). The long chain of hormone-dependent behaviors on the part of both genders helps to guarantee behavioral specificity. In a wide variety of species, courtship behaviors are arranged as described to form a hormone-dependent behavioral funnel, ensuring that reproductively competent conspecifics and only they will end up together.

2. Courtship Behaviors Using Vestibulospinal and Reticulospinal Tracts

Most exquisitely, the nature of courtship behaviors in female rats tips us off to the possibility that the performance of these behaviors themselves, under the influence of estrogen or progesterone, actually prepares the way for lordosis behavior (figures 6.11 and 6.12; figure 7.10). The most abstract way of summarizing all the data available is to say that hormone-dependent behavioral states foster subsequent hormone-dependent behavioral acts. Again, these behaviors are set up as a hormone-dependent behavioral funnel. In general terms, for example, in the female rat, courtship responses include the acceleration of hopping and

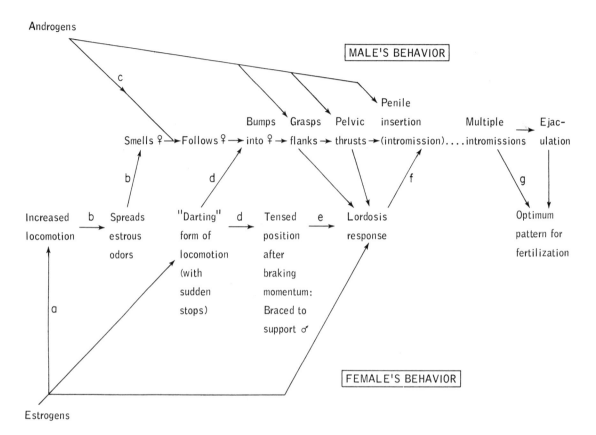

Figure 6.9   Flow chart of events in rat mating behavior, giving a brief summary of how endocrine secretions and behavioral determinants synchronize behavior between the male and
the female to ensure reproduction. Not only do responses by the female allow subsequent responses by the male and vice versa but, even within a gender, foregoing responses can facilitate the performance of later responses. Time reads from left to right. Odor-spreading
behavior of the female (far left) may occur on the night before ovulation, whereas most of
the events on the right occur on the night of ovulation. Small letters refer to notes and references in the original article. (From Pfaff et al., 1972.)

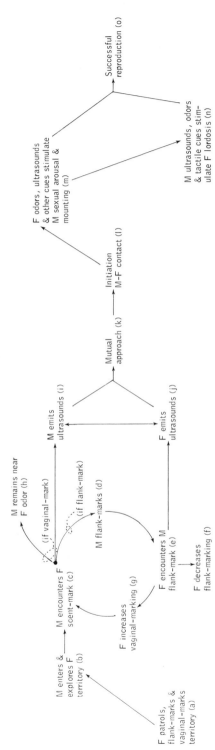

Figure 6.10 Summary of data describing a hormone-dependent chain of social communications leading to reproduction in golden hamsters. Male behavior (M) on top; female behavior (F) on bottom. Communications begin (on the left) with odor marking, in which stimuli are diffuse in time and space. Animals move on (middle of the figure) to ultrasounds, brief and distributed narrowly in space. They finish with tactile communication (right extreme), restricted both in time and in space. Lowercase letters in parentheses code behavior elements for discussion in the text of the original article. Many of the links in this chain of behaviors depend on gonadal hormones. In particular, testosterone facilitates male responses at least at points d, h, m, and o. Estrogens and progestins facilitate female responses at least at points a, g, j, k, n and o. (From Floody & Pfaff, 1977.)

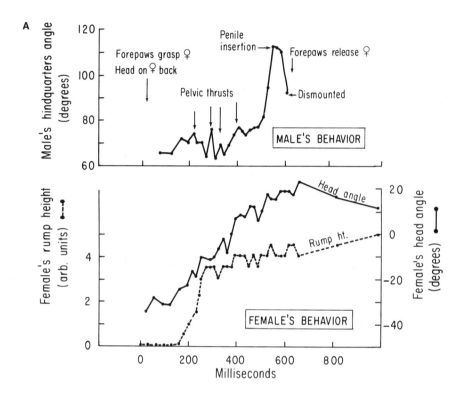

Figure 6.11   Lordosis behavior graphed quantitatively as a sequence of reflexes in the female rat, matched to corresponding responses by the male. (*A*) An individual mating encounter quantified from frame-by-frame analyses of films taken from the side view. In measurements of female rat head angle, 0 degrees is horizontal and head elevation is a change toward more positive numbers. In male rat hindquarters angle measurements, 90 degrees is vertical and a forward thrust is shown by a change toward higher numbers. After flank stimulation of the female by the male's forepaws, initial pelvic thrusts stimulate a full lordosis response which, in turn, allows penile penetration and eventual fertilization. (From Pfaff & Lewis, 1974.) (*B*) A generalized summary of this behavior, showing a flow chart of male and female responses. Even during this very brief encounter, measured in milliseconds (see *A*), responses by the female facilitate subsequent responses by the male, and vice versa. (From Pfaff et al., 1972.)

B MALE'S BEHAVIOR

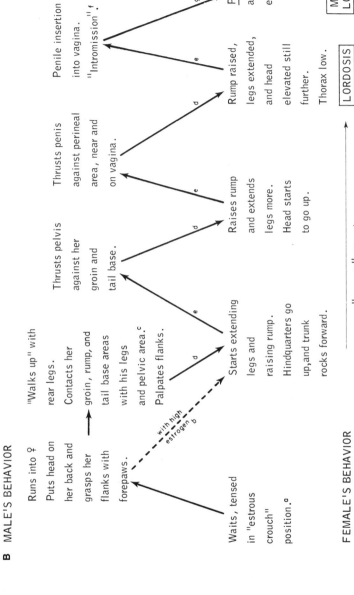

Runs into ♀. Puts head on her back and grasps her flanks with forepaws.

"Walks up" with rear legs. Contacts her groin, rump, and tail base areas with his legs and pelvic area.[c] Palpates flanks.

Thrusts pelvis against her groin and tail base.

Thrusts penis against perineal area, near and on vagina.

Penile insertion into vagina. "Intromission".[f] → Dismount

Starts extending legs and raising rump. Hindquarters go up, and trunk rocks forward.

with high estrogen[b]

Raises rump and extends legs more. Head starts to go up.

Rump raised, legs extended, and head elevated still further. Thorax low.

Peak rump and head elevation.

Waits, tensed in "estrous crouch" position.[a]

"cascade" effect[h]

LORDOSIS

MAXIMUM LORDOSIS

FEMALE'S BEHAVIOR

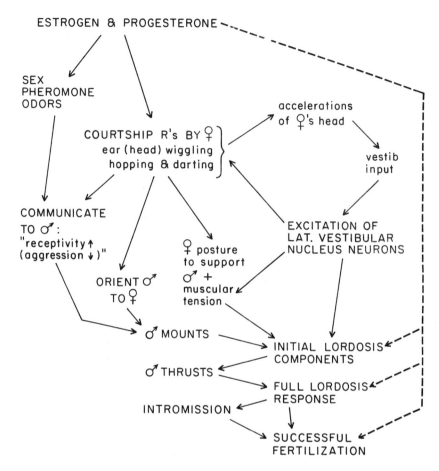

Figure 6.12   A picture of the roles of estrogen and progesterone in preparing neural circuitry so that lordosis behavior eventually can occur. Such preparations include prior displays of courtship (proceptive) behaviors by the female, which cause lateral vestibulospinal excitation and postural tension, which in turn set the stage for lordosis. (From Pfaff, 1980.)

darting and rapid head movements involved in head wiggling, which reflects a high state of excitation in axial motor systems. Notably, these very acts stimulate the vestibular organs by accelerations that produce an even higher pitch of excitation in the lateral vestibulospinal system (references in Pfaff, 1980). This causal sequence comprises a positive feedback system: from vestibulospinal excitation to the head and body musculature that produces the courtship response, to still further vestibulospinal stimulation produced by the courtship response, to further vestibulospinal excitation, and so on. All this excitation stimulates the descending neural pathways and axial muscle systems, which help to guarantee that lordosis behavior will occur (Pfaff, 1980, p. 228).

Saying the same thing in more detailed terms, the electrophysiological and neuroanatomical properties of the lateral vestibulospinal and lateral reticulospinal tracts suit themselves perfectly not only to the facilitation of courtship behaviors and lordosis behavior but to the preparation of the system by courtship behaviors for the eventual lordosis behavior (Pfaff, 1980). Anatomically, the large number of descending connections from these two systems across different spinal levels bilaterally renders them well suited for the governance of behaviors that involve large numbers of axial muscles. Neurophysiologically, the predominant facilitatory effect of the lateral vestibulospinal system is on extensor muscles (Grillner et al., 1970, 1971; Hongo et al., 1975; Lund & Pompeiano, 1968; Ten-Bruggencate & Lundberg, 1974; Wilson, 1975; Wilson et al., 1970; Wilson & Yoshida, 1969). Thus, proceptive behaviors that stimulate the lateral vestibulospinal system will prime the animal for a lordosis reflex that involves vertebral dorsiflexion (i.e., extension).

In addition, the medullary reticulospinal system involves terminations on both sides of the spinal cord at many vertebral levels. Therefore, courtship behaviors that excite the medullary reticulospinal neurons render the animal posturally taut (in the so-called estrous crouch) and ready to perform lordosis. In fact, electrical stimulation of the medullary reticular formation facilitates medial longissimus motoneuron response to dorsal root stimulation, thus elevating responses in a muscle required for lordosis (Brink et al., 1980; Brink & Pfaff, 1979).

Thus, these two descending tracts might have either of two modes of action in facilitating lordosis. One is a preparatory, tonic mode in which spinal circuits relevant for lordosis are prepared for reflex execution before the adequate peripheral stimuli even begin. The second mode of action is what we ordinarily expect from the lordosis circuitry, a hypothalamically enhanced spinobulbospinal reflex loop.

Several lines of evidence presented in this book and previously (Pfaff, 1980) favor the notion that an important mode of action by both lateral vestibulospinal and reticulospinal tracts has a tonic, preparatory component. Before lordosis, in the vicinity of a male rat, highly receptive female rats well primed with estrogen and progesterone may show a highly unusual pattern of locomotion (hopping and darting) and sudden head movements that result in ear wiggling. In fact, in electrophysiological studies, estrous hormones have been shown to enhance rhythmic motor system discharges in correlation with stepping movements (Smith, 1997). The darting form of locomotion consists of sudden bursts of forward movement followed by sudden stops. The sudden stops promote successful male–female mating encounters (Pfaff et al., 1972), first by increasing the chance that the male following from the rear will bump into the female and second by putting the female in a bilaterally balanced posture prepared to support the downward and forward impact of the male's weight. Most importantly, the sudden darts and stops leave the female in a state of muscular tension that facilitates lordosis (Pfaff et al., 1972). The mechanism by which these courtship behaviors (hopping and darting and ear wiggling) facilitate lordosis now can be understood in terms of the electrophysiological features of the lateral vestibulospinal system.

Hopping and darting are composed of unusual linear accelerations along the longitudinal and vertical axes. An important note is that linear acceleration is a stimulus sufficient for exciting electrical action potentials in primary sensory neurons from the otolith of the labyrinth and that the lateral vestibular nucleus itself receives utricular afferents (Brodal et al., 1962; Sato et al., 1996, 1997). Thus, linear acceleration during hopping and darting can stimulate the lateral vestibulospinal system and, in a tonic manner, can facilitate lordosis by increasing the background activity in this system.

The ear wiggling component of courtship behavior of female rats is a function of rapidly alternating head movements (Beach, 1942). Now evident from slow-motion movie film analyses of mating encounters is that ear wiggling results from rapid oscillations of the head around the longitudinal axis (Pfaff & Modianos, 1980). Such stimulation strongly excites the anterior and posterior semicircular canals of the labyrinth (Mountcastle, 1974, 1980), which in turn send primary afferent fibers to the lateral vestibular nucleus. Indeed, Peterson (1970) found that head tilting results in strong excitatory postsynaptic potentials in many cells of the LVN, including those that send efferents, descending outputs, to the spinal cord. Moreover, labyrinthine stimulation can produce excitatory postsynaptic potentials in extensor motoneurons of the spinal cord (Hassen & Barnes, 1975; Wilson et al., 1970). In particular, these anterior semicircular canals have a special role in exciting those Deiters neurons whose axons travel through the lateral vestibulospinal tract (Wilson, 1975; Wilson & Melville-Jones, 1979). This role is especially important because (1) such Deiters neurons are known to have excitatory actions on spinal motor neurons involved in vertebral dorsiflexion, (2) their axons, running through the lateral vestibulospinal tract, can reach the lumbosacral spinal cord, and (3) the lateral vestibulospinal tract is known to be important for lordosis. In fact, stimulation of the anterior semicircular canals actually can cause an upward head movement (Suzuki & Cohen, 1964) like that of lordosis, indicating how this kind of vestibular stimulation during courtship behavior actually could predispose the female rat toward this behavior.

In general, female rat courtship behaviors (e.g., hopping, darting, and ear wiggling) display an unusually high state of excitation of musculature, facilitated by the lateral vestibulospinal system just prior to lordosis. In turn, the vestibular stimulation resulting from these courtship behaviors should lead to an even higher pitch of excitation in the lateral vestibulospinal system and the axial musculature stimulated by it. Thus, these courtship behaviors reveal an adaptive positive feedback relationship in the loop involving the lateral vestibulospinal system, axial musculature, and vestibular input. The excitation of vestibulospinal and axial musculature systems maintained by this positive feedback does not cause lordosis by itself. Instead, it *prepares the animal for successful lordosis* by maintaining high levels of excitation in lordosis-relevant systems. With toni-cally elevated activity in those spinal circuits important for lordosis (i.e., with the appropriate spinal circuits thus prepared), sensory input from adequate cu-taneous stimulation by the male can cause a convincing lordosis response.

C. ENVIRONMENTAL LIMITATIONS ON THE CIRCUIT THAT SATISFY BIOLOGICAL AXIOMS

1. BIOLOGICAL REQUIREMENTS IMPOSED

Even in the simplest animals, sex behavior cannot be driven solely by hormones and the presence of a mate. So far, what we have explained is exactly how par-ticular environmental stimuli—from the male of the species—yield neuronal signals that, through the neural circuit we have analyzed, can be facilitated by sex hormones to yield a specific behavior: lordosis behavior. But, really, a wide range of environmental conditions affect whether reproduction makes sense bi-ologically. Such signals, carrying environmental information from the cell sur-face, can interact with steroid hormones in pathways involving, for example, noradrenergic receptors and G proteins (chapter 7, figure 7.13). How do we view this area of work in a systematic way?

The field of neurobiology contains no universal mathematical equations succinctly expressing a broad range of experimental results. Therefore, as al-gebra and calculus are not going to help us, we must turn to geometry. The safest theoretical approach for the modern neurobiologist is to start from *ax-iomatic* requirements for biologically adaptive neural mechanisms (in our case, for reproduction). An axiom is a statement that is obvious and need not be proved. It is *axiomatic* that if environmental conditions are not appropriate for reproduction, the species will not survive. As we deal only with species that have survived, obviously, brain mechanisms have yielded appropriate behav-ioral responses.

What are the environmental conditions to which the biologically adap-tive brain of a reproducing animal must attend? A broad review has been pro-

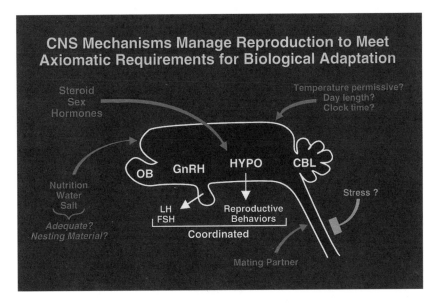

Figure 6.13 (For a color reproduction of this figure, see plate 2.) Because of the high biological cost of reproduction to females, the brain must manage reproductive physiology and behavior in a manner that obeys obvious biological requirements. Several environmental factors (in green) must be present within defined ranges, and stress (in red) must be minimized or it will block reproduction. As a result of neural activity in gonadotropin-releasing hormone (GnRH) neurons and in other hypothalamic (HYPO) cells, release of gonadotropins luteinizing hormone, follicle-stimulating hormone (LH and FSH) from the pituitary is beautifully coordinated with female reproductive behavior. We have figured out the circuitry by which steroid sex hormones in the female potentiate the behavioral effects of stimuli from the male mating partner (in green). Now we are working on how other environmental factors modulate this system. (OB, olfactory bulb; CBL, cerebellum.)

vided by Frank Bronson (1989) and his colleagues. Even the briefest sketch of environmental components that bear on reproductive efficacy yields a list that would keep neurobiologists busy for decades. Many factors must be optimized: food supply, water supply, salt balance, environmental temperature, day length, time of day, absence of stress, and presence of adequate nesting materials, in addition to the simple stimuli from the presence of a mating partner (which we have already analyzed) (figure 6.13). A productive strategy has been to start from the simple circuit we have already discovered and to figure out how a range of environmental conditions, operating through nerve cells and molecular mechanisms, influence reproductive hormones and behavior.

2. TRANSCRIPTION FACTORS COOPERATE AND COMPETE, CONSTITUTING A NEW LEVEL OF NEURAL INTEGRATION

Recently, we saw how stress, especially from cold temperature, can turn off reproduction. For example, the very gene for the nervous system peptide gonadotropin-releasing hormone (GnRH; also known as luteinizing hormone–releasing hormone) can be turned off by glucocorticoid hormones secreted by the adrenal glands, which indicate stress (figure 6.14).

Changes in thyroid hormones indicating unacceptable environmental cold could be important inhibitors of reproduction, especially in small mammals, which have high surface-volume ratios. Thyroid hormones bound to their specific receptors in the cell nucleus can interfere with estrogen receptors binding to the same portions of DNA. As documented in detail in chapter 7, and demonstrated in our laboratory, Yuan-Shan Zhu has shown that thyroid hormones can interfere with estrogen-stimulated gene expression in the brain. In turn, Tammy Dellovade found that thyroid hormones can interfere with estrogen-stimulated lordosis behavior (see chapter 7, figure 10). Because elevated thyroid hormone levels signal environmental cold, our experiment offers the possibility of exploring ethological facts at a molecular level.

New work with TR gene knockout mice in our lab (Dellovade et al., submitted) shows that thyroid interference depends on the gene for TR-β. Thus we

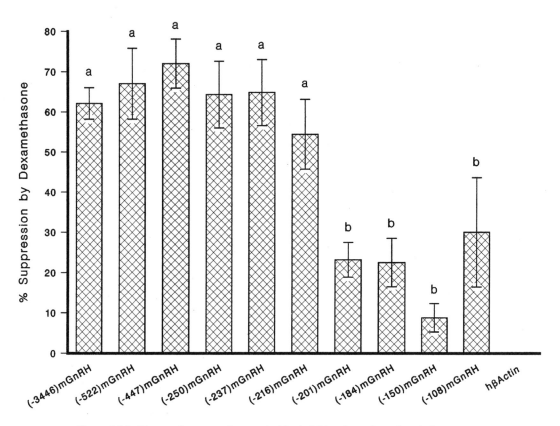

Figure 6.14   Dexamethasone, a glucocorticoid mimicking the action of cortisol, suppresses transcriptional activity of specific portions of the promoter for the gonadotropin-releasing hormone (GnRH) gene. In a set of serial promoter deletions, the glucocorticoid action to suppress GnRH transcription was large up until the point that the promoter was deleted down to −201 bases (bars marked *a* compared to bars marked *b*). (From Chandran et al., 1996.)

can say that the TR-β gene operates on lordosis by blocking ER functions (see also chapter 7). More generally, this work (now including zoological, DNA-binding, transcriptional, and behavioral data) makes use of hormone-triggered mechanisms to show how nuclear hormone receptor interactions on the surface of DNA may offer a new level of neural integration (figure 6.15)

The principle illustrated here is that transcription factors, such as estrogen receptors and thyroid receptors, can cooperate and compete with one another, thus integrating signals that influence behavior. Four levels of neuronal integration include morphological, electrical, neurochemical, and (now) genomic.

D. Smell

1. Electrical and Behavioral Responses to Pheromones

The primary role of the forebrain module for lordosis behavior is inhibitory: Damaging the preoptic area or the septum or most of the amygdala actually will improve lordosis behavior performance. A possible exception to this generalization has to do with roles for smells in reproductive physiology.

Natural smells from plants, animals, or (indeed) human beings often are called *pheromones.* Smells such as pheromones let animals know when the situation is right for mating (e.g., signaling the abundance of food, the availability of mating partners, etc.). Mice provide wonderful examples of the effects of odors on reproductive physiology: Females can be brought into puberty faster by the smells of males, their estrous cycles can be altered, and their pregnancy can be affected. Humans too can be affected thus. In college dormitories, a woman's menstrual cycle can be affected by those around her (McClintock, 1971). Compounds emanating from women in the late follicular phase of their

Figure 6.15 Schematic illustration of how nerve cell nuclear proteins other than the estrogen receptor (ER) itself could help to account for sexual dimorphisms (*top*) in neuronal genetic regulation, as well as for brain regional differences (*bottom*). (From Pfaff et al., 1996.)

Genetic sex specificity, theory

Genetic ♀   · Genetic ♂

a. Associated protein required

b. Competing protein interferes

c. Squelching protein

d. Promoter access

Tissue specificity, theory

Ventromedial hypothal.   Amygdala

e. Associated protein required

f. Competing protein interferes

g. Squelching protein

h. Promoter access

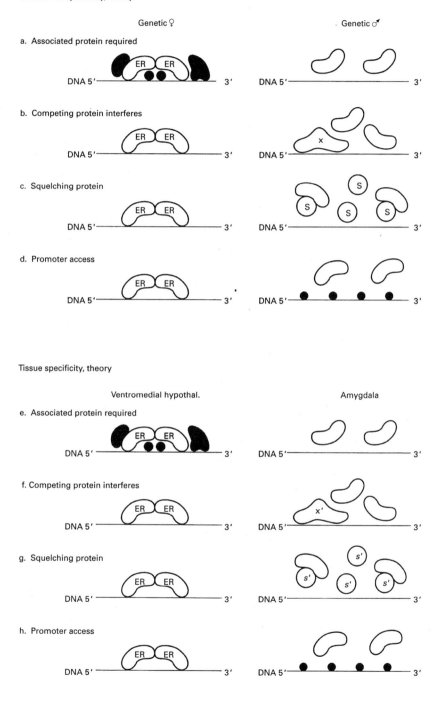

menstrual cycles accelerated the ovulatory surge of luteinizing hormone of recipient women, whereas compounds from the same donors collected later in
the menstrual cycle delayed the surge (Stern & McClintock, 1998).

Experiments on lower animal brains and behaviors have provided the
greatest insights because of the ability to perform experiments on cellular mechanisms. Recording of electrophysiological responses to natural odors clearly established that male rodent forebrain neurons respond strongly to odors from the
female rodent. Hamsters are so primitive—in the respect that few experiential
factors bear on this type of behavior—that even if they have not been exposed
to female odors since they were weaned from their mother, they will prefer the
odor of an estrous female hamster (figure 6.16). In addition, the female can respond to odors from other animals. Not all these chemosensory signals come
through the olfactory system proper. New biophysical results show interesting
electrophysiological responses to pheromones, mediated by the vomeronasal
organ, a specialized cigar-shaped tube of chemically sensitive tissue at the very
base of the olfactory apparatus, just above the roof of the mouth (Moss et al.,
1997). Presumably, responses of the vomeronasal-accessory olfactory system
underlie the dramatic stimulation of mating behavior often seen in these laboratory rodents.

Females actually can learn and perform arbitrarily chosen responses to
gain access to the male, partly by using odors as cues (J. Matthews et al., unpublished observations). In fact, in rare instances, the odor of the male by itself
can trigger the mating posture in a female hamster.

2. CLONING OF OLFACTORY AND VOMERONASAL "RECEPTOR" GENES

Two recent discoveries will blast open the field of olfactory signaling and help
us to figure out how odors control reproductive drives in animals and human
beings. The first discovery that will help this field of work greatly has to do
with olfactory signaling itself. Until recently, we did not know exactly what olfactory receptor molecules are. Then Linda Buck and Richard Axel, working

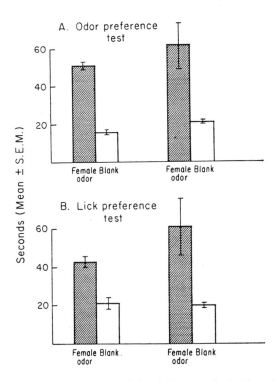

Figure 6.16 On systematic testing, even adult male hamsters that had been isolated from females and their odors since the time of weaning showed significant preferences for female odors. Group B males, isolated in this way, showed preferences just as strong as those of group A males, which had been preexposed to females. This conclusion applied both during odor preference tests (measurements of sniffing time) or lick preference tests (utilizing natural male hamster responses). The preferences depended absolutely on the presence of circulating testosterone. (From Gregory et al., 1975.)

at Columbia University, cloned olfactory epithelium genes that appear to code for olfactory receptor proteins: The DNA of these genes gives rise to synthesized messenger RNAs that in turn code for proteins on the cell surface, which themselves recognize odors (Buck, 1996).

An even more surprising development emerged when Dulac and Axel (1995) compared genes expressed in the vomeronasal organ to those in the olfactory system proper. Expecting that the two sets of receptors would be similar, they were astounded to find that olfactory receptor–like proteins were by and large not expressed in the vomeronasal organ. Instead, Dulac has reported six families of receptor proteins quite separate from those in the olfactory system proper (Dulac & Axel, 1995). Now, biophysical recordings must confirm that these gene products actually are receptors.

Olfactory and vomeronasal receptors, stimulating consequent behavioral responses, remind us of the differences between the types of behavioral changes explained here and those that have been emphasized throughout most of twentieth century neurophysiology. Because most people have been impressed by the ability of the human brain to store new information, the ideas of learning and memory have been dominated by studies of visual and auditory inputs, with an emphasis on formal learning tasks. Remember that Apollo was the Greek god of the sun. So far, twentieth century neurophysiology has been dominated by an Apollonian type of neurobiology. Dionysus was the Greek god of desire. Smell-driven behaviors, dependent on sex hormones, partake of a Dionysian form of neurobiology. It just so happens that this latter type of neural function is necessary for reproduction. Tying together sex hormones and smell, Getchell et al. (1996) recently reported immunoreactivity for estrogen receptors in vomeronasal and olfactory receptors, so hormone-influenced neuroplasticity could occur at a very early stage of olfactory processing.

Is the sort of forebrain circuitry coming from the olfactory and vomeronasal systems important for human feelings and behavior? It must be, for if it were not, no perfume industry would exist. Is it any accident that the notes for this part of the book were written in the perfume section of a department store?

---

3. MIGRATION OF NEURONS WHICH MAKE THE PROTEIN GOVERNING SEX, FROM THE OLFACTORY PIT TO THE FOREBRAIN

The nerve cells that govern reproduction (i.e., neurons that manufacture GnRH) actually migrate from the developing olfactory pit in the embryo to the basal forebrain (Schwanzel-Fukuda & Pfaff, 1989). This process has been demonstrated in zoological forms as relatively simple (in the standard phylogenetic tree) as fish and as complex as human beings (Schwanzel-Fukuda et al., 1996; figure 6.17). In fact, failure of this migration is associated with failure of *libido* in men (see chapter 8; Schwanzel-Fukuda et al., 1989b). Mechanisms underlying the GnRH neuronal migration from the nose into the brain have been investigated in considerable detail (figure 6.18).

Once GnRH neurons arrive in the preoptic area, they collect an impressive array of chemical inputs consistent with the large number of signals required (axiomatically) to manage reproduction successfully in all its endocrine and behavioral aspects.

E. SUMMARY

The work reviewed in this chapter demonstrates that natural biochemicals under our experimental control act in specific parts of the central nervous system to cause a particular behavior. By inference, the principle is established, therefore, that mammalian behavior is determinable. Specific hormonal inputs and sensory signals are shown to interact in a well-studied, specific neural circuit that includes the midbrain and hypothalamus and, thus, to allow the performance of an integrated reproductive behavior. The foregoing behaviors that comprise courtship exquisitely prepare the established neural circuit for the performance of lordosis behavior. Knowing a lot about the circuit and its consequent behavior permits us to unite zoological and environmental thinking with molecular methodology. The result is that we see how internal and external signals combine to influence reproductive behavior; we see also how transcription factors can interact in neurons in the service of neural integration. Now possi-

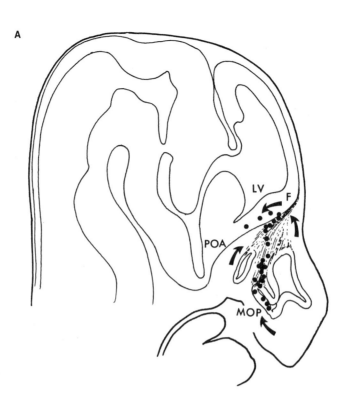

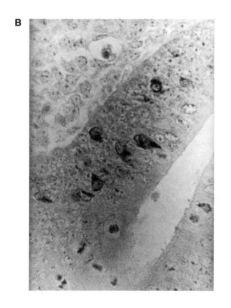

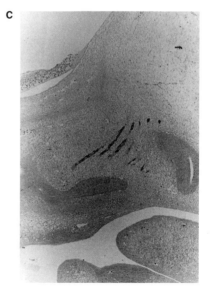

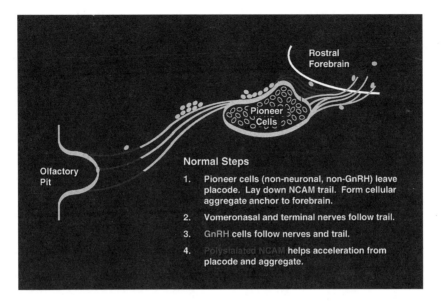

Figure 6.18   (For a color reproduction of this figure, see plate 4.) Schematic summary of steps involved in the migration of newly born gonadotropin-releasing hormone neurons (red ovals) from the olfactory pit into the developing basal forebrain. This migration, established by the discovery of Schwanzel-Fukuda and Pfaff (1989), occurs in all vertebrates studied and is essential for the development of neural controls over reproduction. Participation by neural cell adhesion molecule (NCAM) is shown using color coding. Additional reading includes papers on NCAM and on human brain development (Schwanzel-Fukuda et al., 1992, 1994, 1996).

◀ Figure 6.17   (For a color reproduction of this figure, see plate 3.) (*A*) Tracing of gonadotropin-releasing hormone (GnRH) neurons (black dots) migrating along the route from the medial side of the olfactory placode (MOP) up the nose, into the basal forebrain (F) below the lateral ventricle (LV), and toward the preoptic area (POA). The migration starts on days 10 and 11 during embryonic mouse development and is largely complete by day 16. (Data from Schwanzel-Fukuda & Pfaff, 1989.) (*B*) At high magnification, immunocytochemically stained GnRH neurons in the olfactory placode of the embryonic mouse. GnRH-expressing neurons were recognized using the antibody LR1. (*C*) A photomicrograph taken at lower magnification than in *B* and at a slightly later stage of development, showing "trains" of GnRH neurons migrating across the olfactory apparatus from the olfactory placode (near the bottom) toward the basal forebrain (f, near the top). GnRH neurons tend to migrate in clusters. (From Schwanzel-Fukuda & Pfaff, 1989.)

ble is an understanding of how interactions of internal and external signals, including interactions among transcription factors, help the organism to satisfy the biologically axiomatic requirements for sensible reproductive behavior.

The steroid sex hormones involved here actually employ changes in gene expression that lead to hormone-influenced behavioral end points, as illustrated in chapter 7. In turn, we see both direct and indirect effects of gene products on mammalian behaviors.

7

GENETIC INFLUENCES ON HORMONE-CONTROLLED DRIVE

The apple never falls far from the tree.

In this chapter, we learn that such steroid sex hormones as estrogens and progestins influence the expression of certain genes in nerve cells in those specific
parts of the brain that control sexual behavior performance (part A). In turn,
the products of those genes facilitate lordosis behavior and related reproductive behaviors typical of females in the laboratory animals studied (part B).
Conversely, inherited genetic states in animals or humans (including sex differences) demonstrate roles for genetic influences on sexual motivation (chapter section B.2).

A. SEX HORMONE EFFECTS ON GENES IN THE BRAIN

Hormones influence genes, and those gene products influence behavior (see for example, figure 5.13). Therefore, it is most efficient to conclude that part of
the way in which those hormones influence behavior is through genetic alterations. Different genes are turned on by estrogens in different neurons, and
their respective gene products have different biochemical functions within those
neurons.

1. PROGESTERONE RECEPTOR

Perhaps one of the best examples of the foregoing "syllogism" is the effect of estrogen on the gene for the progesterone receptor (PR) (figure 7.1). Not only does estrogen injection induce the binding of radioactive progesterone in the hypothalamus; it causes an increase in the messenger RNA for the progesterone receptor (Romano et al., 1989a). This effect occurs in females but not males and is restricted to brain regions related to reproductive behaviors (Lauber et al., 1991). The effect of estrogen actually is transcriptional (figure 7.2), as shown by the use of neurotropic viral vectors for in vivo promoter analysis, a technique in which the ability of the PR gene promoter to respond is tested in normal neurons (Scott, 1996 and unpublished data). Most exciting, estrogen induces PR in the very cells in the hypothalamus needed for reproductive behavior. *Because PR itself is a genetic transcription factor, these experiments represent the first example of the induction of a specific transcription factor key for the performance of a specific behavior (Romano et al., 1989a).* Both antisense DNA (Ogawa et al., 1994) and genetic knockout technology (Lydon et al., 1995; Ogawa et al.,

Figure 7.1   A wealth of information supports the hypothesis that progesterone binds to progesterone receptor (PR) in hypothalamic neurons, inducing new genes whose products help to mediate progesterone's effects on female reproductive behavior. Particularly important is the discovery of the PR-B form of messenger RNA, for facilitation of transcription in hypothalamic neurons, as opposed to the PR-A form, which would be expected to block transcription. Detailed evidence has been provided with respect to the estrogen induction of PR (middle column) and with respect to sex differences in progesterone receptor induction and behavior (right column). Studies have been completed with respect to PR itself (top row), the involvement of its gene (middle row), and the participation of PR in the ventromedial hypothalamus (bottom row). *Superscripts refer to literature references as follows:* [1]Ogawa et al., 1994; [2]Brown & Blaustein, 1984 and Vathy et al; [3]Romano et al., 1989; [3a]MacClusky & McEwen, 1980; [4]Parsons et al., 1991, and Lauber et al., 1991; [5]Scott et al., unpublished data; [6]Scott et al., 1997; [7]Scott et al., unpublished data; [8]Lydon et al., 1995, and Ogawa et al., 1998, in preparation; [9]Glaser & Barfield, 1984, and Pleim et al., 1989; [10]Krebs et al., 1997; [10a]Scott et al., unpublished data; [11]Parsons et al.; [12]Scott et al., unpublished data; [13]Parsons et al., and Scott et al., unpublished data; [14]Parsons et al., 1980, 1982a, b; [15]Lauber et al., 1991.

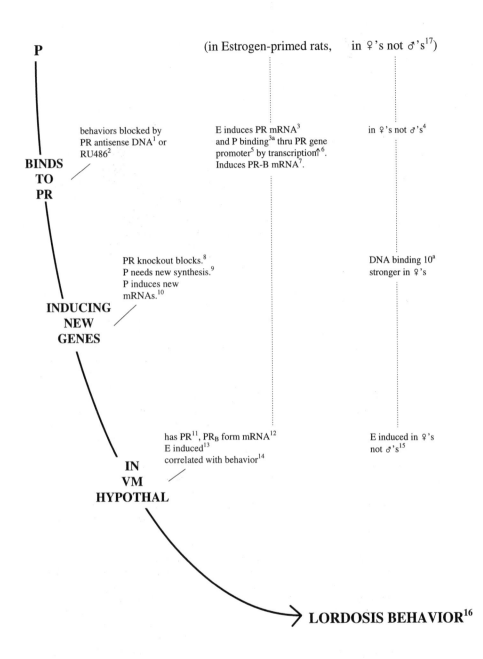

P

(in Estrogen-primed rats,   in ♀'s not ♂'s[17])

**BINDS
TO
PR**

behaviors blocked by
PR antisense DNA[1] or
RU486[2]

E induces PR mRNA[3]
and P binding[3a] thru PR gene
promoter[5] by transcription↑[6].
Induces PR-B mRNA[7].

in ♀'s not ♂'s[4]

**INDUCING
NEW
GENES**

PR knockout blocks.[8]
P needs new synthesis.[9]
P induces new
mRNAs.[10]

DNA binding 10[a]
stronger in ♀'s

**IN
VM
HYPOTHAL**

has PR[11], PR_B form mRNA[12]
E induced[13]
correlated with behavior[14]

E induced in ♀'s
not ♂'s[15]

LORDOSIS BEHAVIOR[16]

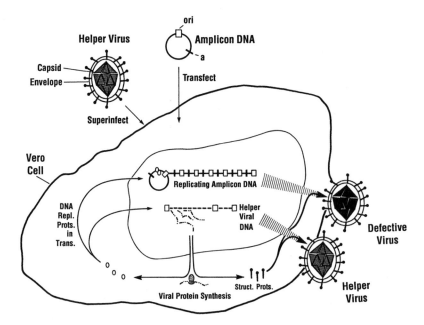

Figure 7.2 (For a color reproduction of this figure, see plate 5.) (*Above*) Method for preparing neurotropic viral vectors from a fragment of the herpes viral genome, used for gene transfer into brain and for in vivo promoter analysis in the central nervous system (from Kaplitt et al., 1993). This method was used for the experiments depicted later in this figure and in figures 7.4 and 7.5, as well as for other experiments in our laboratory (e.g., Kaplitt et al., 1991). First, the DNA of the viral vector itself (the "amplicon") is transfected into a host cell (such as a Vero cell). The next morning, a helper virus—a temperature-sensitive, mutated virus—is superinfected. Both sets of DNA go to the Vero cell nucleus. Only at the permissive temperature (31°C) does the helper virus provide both the proteins needed by the viral vector DNA needs to replicate, in *trans,* and the helper virus provide the protein for the neurotropic protein coat of the vector. The viral vector itself, exiting the Vero cell, is a "defective virus": It is a small bit of the herpes DNA that contains only the origin of replication, the cleavage and packaging sequence, and the genes of interest for the central nervous system experiment (from Kaplitt et al., 1993). (*Opposite*) Use of neurotropic viral vectors (herpes "amplicon") for in vivo promoter analysis. Here we ask, *in the context of normal pituitary nuclear proteins (top, A–D) or normal hypothalamic nuclear proteins (bottom),* two questions: First, can a selected portion of the progesterone receptor promote drive transcription of a reporter gene (β-galactosidase) in appropriate pituitary or hypothalamic cells, respectively? Second, can estradiol regulate transcription of the reporter gene through the progesterone receptor promoter in those cells? (*Top, A*) Low-power photomicrograph of the rat pituitary taken from an estrogen-treated female. Note the widespread and dense expression of β-galactosidase in the anterior pituitary. As a built-in anatomical control, the posterior pituitary shows no expression of the reporter gene under this promoter. (*Top, B*) High-power photomicrograph from an estrogen-treated anterior pituitary. Dense cellular expression of the reporter gene stimulated by estrogen action through the progesterone receptor promoter is evident. (*Top, C*) In the control, vehicle-treated female rat anterior pituitary, only weak reporter gene expression is seen. (*Top, D*) As an additional viral control, when only the helper virus (without the viral vector) was injected into the sella turcica, no cells are stained. (From Scott et al. *Molecular Brain Research,* submitted, 1999). (*Bottom, A*) Ventromedial hypothalamic neurons showed significant levels of reporter gene expression stimulated by estrogen working through the progesterone receptor promoter. Every blue-green cell body seen here indicates robust progesterone receptor activity in hypothalamic

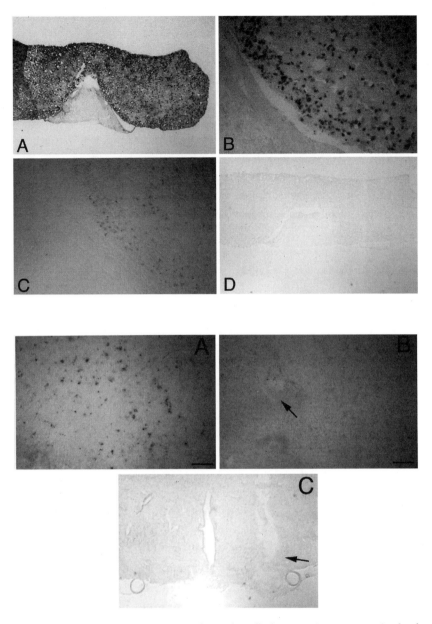

neurons sampled from an estrogen-treated rat. The cells demonstrating estrogen-stimulated progesterone receptor promoter activity include the very neurons through which estrogen acts to turn on the progesterone receptor itself and lordosis behavior. (*Bottom, B*) In a control, ovariectomized female rat, hardly any reporter gene–expressing cells were seen in the medial hypothalamus, even near the viral vector injection site (arrow). (*Bottom, C*) When hypothalamic tissue was injected with the control helper virus only (no viral vector included), no staining was seen. (From Scott et al., 1998.)

1997) show that gene expression for PR is, in its turn, necessary for normal hormone-driven reproductive behavior.

The viral vector evidence, in which the PR genetic promoter is attached to a "reporter gene"—β-galactosidase—is striking. It shows that estrogen induces PR gene expression in pituitary and hypothalamus (see figure 7.2). Further, it demonstrates that the estrogen effect is transcriptional, working through a specific part of the PR gene promoter.

These findings establish the principle that a hormone (estrogen) working through a transcription factor (estrogen receptor) can induce expression of another transcription factor gene (PR) in the brain, the action of which in those neurons is necessary for a behavior.

2. THE OPIOID PEPTIDE GENE PREPROENKEPHALIN

Likewise, estrogen induces expression of the gene for the opioid peptide enkephalin (Romano et al., 1988), the messenger RNA of which is correlated perfectly with the performance of female rat reproductive behavior (Lauber et al., 1990a). In the ventromedial hypothalamus (VMH), enkephalin messenger RNA fluctuates during the normal estrus cycle (Funabashi et al., 1995). Antisense DNA evidence (Nicot et al., 1997) strongly suggests that something about enkephalin gene expression is important for the performance of lordosis (figure 7.3). Again, the use of a viral vector for in vivo promoter analysis shows not only that the enkephalin gene promoter directs expression of a reporter gene correctly in the brain (figure 7.4) but that it is turned on by estrogen (figure 7.5) (Kaplitt et al., 1994; Yin et al., 1994). Because the normal receptor, the delta opioid receptor, for enkephalin is increased also by estradiol (Quiñones-Jenab et al., unpublished data), the enkephalin effect and the receptor effect multiply each other. Again, the parallels between gene expression and behavior are striking: Enkephalin induction occurs in females much more efficiently than in males and is strongest in the parts of the brain correlated with female reproductive behavior (see figure 7.3).

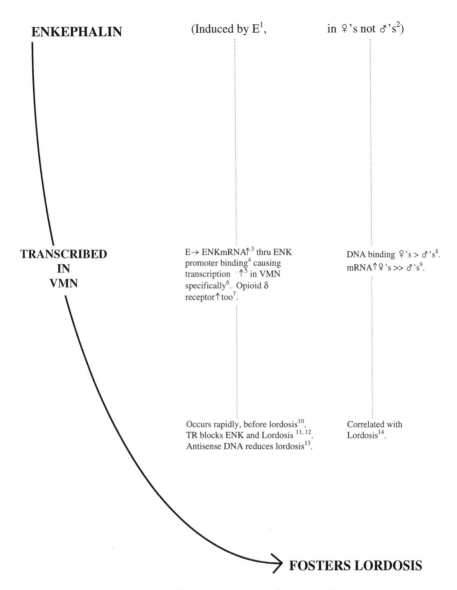

ENKEPHALIN   (Induced by E^1,   in ♀'s not ♂'s^2)

TRANSCRIBED IN VMN

E→ ENKmRNA↑^{3} thru ENK promoter binding^4 causing transcription ↑^{5} in VMN specifically^6. Opioid δ receptor↑too^7.

DNA binding ♀'s > ♂'s^8. mRNA↑♀'s >> ♂'s^9.

Occurs rapidly, before lordosis^{10}. TR blocks ENK and Lordosis $^{11, 12}$. Antisense DNA reduces lordosis^{13}.

Correlated with Lordosis^{14}.

FOSTERS LORDOSIS

Figure 7.3   A large amount of information supports the hypothesis that the gene for the opi-oid peptide enkephalin is transcribed in the ventromedial hypothalamic nucleus (VMN) and that its product is important for estrogenic effects on female reproductive behavior. Major re-sults include its induction by estrogen (E, middle column), and its sexual differentiation (right column). Mechanisms related to transcriptional control (middle row) and temporal features of messenger RNA induction (bottom row) support the overall picture. *Suprascripts refer to litera-ture references as follows:* [1]Romano et al., 1988; [2]Romano et al., 1990; [3]Romano et al., 1988; [4]Zhu & Pfaff, 1995; [5]Zhu, unpublished data, and Yin et al., 1994; [6]Romano et al., 1988; [7]Quiñones-Jenab et al., 1996; [8]Zhu et al., 1995, unpublished data; [9]Romano et al., 1990; [10]Zhu et al., unpublished data, and Romano et al., 1989; [11]Zhu et al., 1996; [12]Dellovade et al., 1996; [13]Nicot et al., 1997; [14]Lauber et al., 1990.

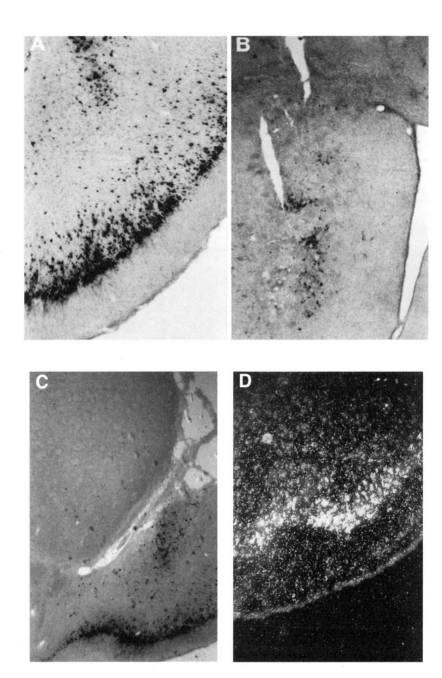

This genomic action of estrogen on enkephalin in VMH neurons appears to produce a partial analgesia (allowing the female to tolerate strong cutaneous and visceral stimuli from the male). VMH projections in the lordosis circuit (see figure 6.1) to ventral periaqueductal gray would be most important in this regard (Bodnar et al., unpublished data).

Multiplicative Actions of Estrogens

In the foregoing case, as in other cases (see chapter 10), estrogens can turn on the genes both for the ligand (the occupant of a receptor) and the receptor itself. Here, the ligand is enkephalin, and the receptor itself is the δ-receptor, both increased by estrogens (Quiñones-Jenab et al., unpublished data; Romano et al., 1988). We have similar examples in which the peptide oxytocin, which fosters affiliative behaviors, is turned on by estrogen, as is the transcription of the oxytocin receptor (Chung et al., 1991; Quiñones-Jenab et al., 1997; Schumacher et al., 1990, 1993). Further, under behaviorally relevant conditions, long-term actions of estrogens can increase the messenger RNA for gonadotropen releasing hormone (GnRH) and can increase the levels of messenger RNA for the

Figure 7.4   (For a color reproduction of this figure, see plate 6.) First use of a viral vector for in vivo promoter analysis in the central nervous system revealed region-specific and cell-specific gene expression (data from Kaplitt et al., 1994). Dr. Michael J. Kaplitt prepared a herpes simplex "amplicon" viral vector, in which 2,700 bases of the rat enkephalin promoter were placed upstream of the bacterial lacZ gene, to drive expression of that reporter gene. Thus, effective transcription through that promoter would yield blue-green nerve cells as against a violet counterstain. This viral vector was microinjected into selected regions of the rat central nervous system. Positive expression, denoted by the blue-green cells, matched endogenous enkephalin expression and is illustrated in the piriform cortex (A) and in the caudate nucleus (B). Control microinjections into regions that do not express enkephalin endogenously did not yield these collections of blue-green cells. Further, fidelity of viral vector–mediated gene expression with respect to the endogenous enkephalin gene's expression was illustrated by the excellent match between the β-galactosidase pattern in the piriform cortex (C) and the pattern shown after in situ hybridization for endogenous enkephalin messenger RNA (D).

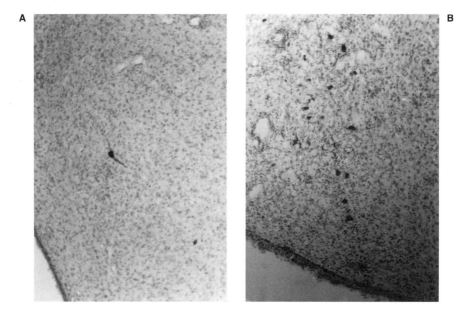

Figure 7.5 (For a color reproduction of this figure, see plate 7.) Use of a neurotropic viral vector (as described in figure 7.4) to demonstrate estrogenic regulation of the enkephalin promoter in medial hypothalamic neurons. Yin and Kaplitt prepared a herpes simplex "amplicon" viral vector in which 2,700 bases of the rat enkephalin promoter were used to drive a β-galactosidase reporter gene. This they microinjected among ventromedial hypothalamic neurons in ovariectomized female rats that then were given either vehicle control (*A*) or were given an injection subcutaneously with estradiol benzoate (*B*). Estrogen treatment clearly increased transcription through the enkephalin promoter, yielding a larger number of blue-green stained cell bodies (Yin et al., 1994, Endocrine Society Abstract and unpublished data). This finding fits with previous results (see text). These data also illustrate the first use in the CNS of a viral vector to demonstrate physiological regulation of a gene promoter.

GnRH receptor (Jennes et al., 1997; Quiñones-Jenab et al., 1996; Roberts et al., 1989; Rosie et al., 1990; Rothfeld et al., 1989). Multiplicative actions of hormones on transcriptional systems would appear to produce changes not only in protein product but especially in physiological activity through those systems, which would be especially important biologically and behaviorally (figure 7.6; also see chapter 10).

In addition, because estrogen increases both the messenger RNA for a peptide ligand (enkephalin) and for its favorite receptor (the δ–opioid receptor), these two effects also could be expected to multiply each other. Similarly, estradiol turns on the gene for the peptide oxytocin in a specific subset of paraventricular hypothalamic neurons and the gene for the oxytocin receptor. Again, these multiplicative, additive, or synergistic effects are likely to be especially clear, biologically and behaviorally.

The data summarized in figures 7.1 through 7.6 show how hormones have been used to turn on genes in the brain at particular times and in particular neuronal groups. In doing so, they bring these genes into the explanation of natural reproductive behaviors.

3. INTERACTIONS AMONG TRANSCRIPTION FACTORS

If researchers were excited by the finding that a ligand-dependent transcription factor, such as the estrogen receptor (ER), could induce another transcription factor, the PR, in the service of reproductive behavior, even more astounding is the notion that such transcription factors as ER and thyroid hormone receptor (TR) can interact with each other in a way that obeys environmental commands and subsequently governs reproductive behavior.

This subject came to our attention when we realized that, at the molecular level, TRs could compete with the DNA binding of ERs to genetic estrogen response elements (EREs) (figure 7.7). This finding is biologically important because environmental cold can increase circulating thyroid hormones and, therefore, the amount of liganded TR in the brain (figure 7.8). After all, the environmental constraints on reproduction in the female are severe

------

Gene Products Elevated by Estrogen (E) in Hypothalamus

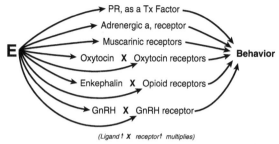

Figure 7.6   Estrogen administration leads to the upregulation of several transcriptional systems in medial hypothalamic neurons. In turn, the products of those genes foster female reproductive behaviors. Therefore, these genomic actions of estradiol are demonstrated to be on the causal route by which estrogens facilitate behavior. Different gene products have different roles. For example, the progesterone receptor (PR) is itself a transcription factor (Tx Factor). Other gene products facilitate specific neurotransmitter or neuropeptide systems. Note that where estrogen administration would upregulate both a ligand and its cognate receptor, the two hormonal effects could multiply.

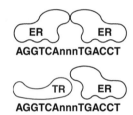

Figure 7.7   On the DNA nucleotide base sequence comprising an estrogen–response element (ERE), competitive binding by a liganded thyroid hormone receptor (TR) could disrupt productive homodimer binding by estrogen receptor (ER). This process is not the only way in which thyroid hormones could have an impact on reproductive behavior, but it does represent a clear mechanism by which environmental disturbances, especially cold temperature, could use molecular alterations to signal important hypothalamic neurons.

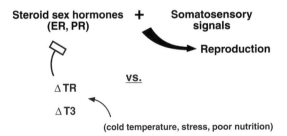

Figure 7.8   The mechanisms by which somatosensory signals and steroid sex hormones integrate to produce reproductive behavior have been worked out in detail. Now, disruptive environmental perturbations, especially cold, can be seen as altering circulating thyroid hormone levels, thus altering liganded thyroid hormone receptor in brain (TR), thus blocking behaviorally important ER effects.

because of the prolonged and expensive biological investment she must make once pregnant (Dellovade et al., 1995). Therefore, environmental signals indicating an entire range of noxious circumstances, such as cold, stress, and inappropriate food supplies, might well be expected to interfere with reproductive processes, including female reproductive behavior. Relations between thyroid hormones and reproductive physiology had been explored to some extent (Dellovade et al., 1995) but, until recently, very little molecular work and no behavioral work had been performed.

Both ERs and TRs can bind to DNA at a sequence wherein "consensus half-site" is AGGTCA. A consensus site on DNA for one of a gene's transcription factors is composed of a particular sequence of nucleotide bases that reliably confers the greatest facilitation of transcription by a given factor. Intriguing is that the nucleotide base sequences conferring sensitivity of gene transcription to ERs and TRs respectively, both include AGGTCA. Thus, TR could compete with ER for occupation of this sequence on a neuronal gene promoter. We have shown that TRs participate in ER-laden complexes in hypothalamic neurons: Purified TR can bind to ER-dependent sequences. In DNA binding experiments, the addition of high-affinity thyroid hormone response elements can draw proteins away from ER complexes. Furthermore, TR-specific antibodies can "supershift" DNA-binding complexes on estrogen-stimulated portions of gene promoters, changing the mass of the DNA-bound complex, thus revealing the participation of TR in the complex (Zhu et al., 1996; unpublished data). Even more important, estrogen-stimulated transcription is attenuated by liganded TR (Zhu et al., 1996; figure 7.9). This process is not limited to transcription that depends on consensus EREs but is true for the enkephalin ERE important for reproductive behavior (see foregoing). In addition, interruption of ER-dependent transcription can proceed by a mechanism separate from competitive DNA binding, as a mutated TR, which cannot bind normally to DNA, also had this effect (Zhu et al., 1996).

Do these interactions between ER and TR have any behavioral consequences? Experiments used ovariectomized female rats treated with high doses of T_3 or vehicle and revealed that thyroid hormone treatment resulted in lower

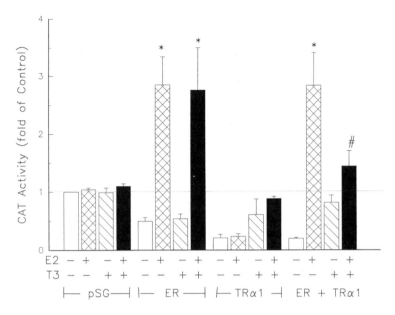

Figure 7.9 Proteins from the thyroid hormone (TR) alpha gene can inhibit estrogen-induced gene transcription in a ligand-dependent manner. In cotransfection experiments using CV-1 cells, the control vector itself (pSG) supported neither estradiol (E2) nor thyroid hormone (T3) effects on transcription (measured by CAT activity). When the estrogen receptor (ER) gene was transfected, E2 stimulated transcription, but T3 had no effect. Conversely, when only a TR gene was transfected, no estrogen effect resulted. In the critical experiment (right side), both ER and TR were transfected into the CV-1 cells. Now, E2 led to a large stimulation of transcription, and coadministration of T3 significantly reduced that transcription. (From Zhu et al., 1996.)

levels of estrogen-dependent lordosis behavior (Dellovade et al., 1996). These same experimental results were extended to female mice (Morgan et al., 1997). Significantly, thyroidectomized ovariectomized females had higher levels of lordosis behavior than did controls, indicating that endogenous thyroid hormones also have this antireproductive effect (figure 7.10). In the manner of control experiments, the evident thyroid hormone interference with estradiol-induced behavior could not be explained by a reduction of concentrations of estradiol in the blood nor by a reduction of estrogen responsiveness throughout the body nor by a reduction of hypothalamic ER immunoreactivity.

Now it is possible to summarize causal routes by which two genes affect lordosis behavior. The ER gene product turns on several transcriptional systems important for lordosis. The TR-β gene blocks ER functions.

The competitive interactions between ER and TR can be extended to other systems. During in situ hybridization studies of oxytocin messenger RNA, Dellovade discovered that estrogen leads to increased oxytocin messenger RNA in a subset of paraventricular hypothalamic (PVN) neurons. The estrogen effect was inhibited by either exogenous or endogenous thyroid hormone; in return, thyroid hormone effects were inhibited by estrogens (figure 7.11; see also figure 10.4). This finding is behaviorally important as oxytocin, working through the estrogen-dependent oxytocin receptor, stimulates a variety of behaviors related to reproduction. Even in the pituitary gland, estrogen-thyroid opposition was apparent. Zhu et al. (1997) found that removal of the ovaries led to weight decreases and RNA decreases in the female pituitary, whereas castration of the male led to increased weight and increased RNA. Estrogen treatment led to a restoration of total pituitary RNA in the female but not the male. The RNA observations were matched by pituitary nuclear proteins that showed a slow mobility complex induced by estrogen in females to a much greater extent than in males. The punch line: The estrogen effect was blocked by concomitant thyroid hormone administration.

The opposition of thyroid hormones to reproductive function may turn out to be a bigger story than first was anticipated. In certain seasonal birds (Bentley et al., 1997; Goldsmith et al. 1984a,b) and in sheep, (Moenter et al.,

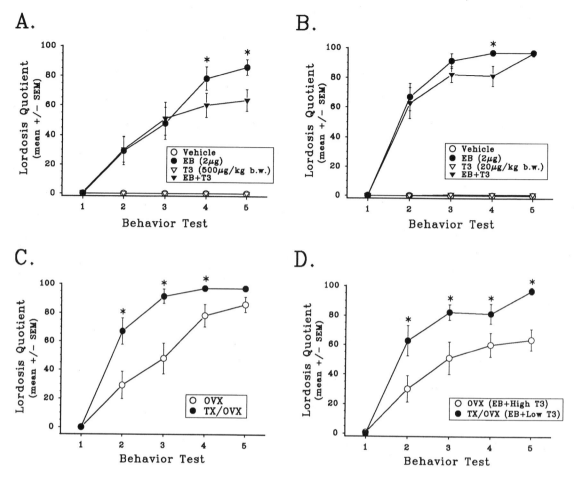

Figure 7.10   Administration of the thyroid hormone (T3) caused a lower reproductive behavior response to estradiol treatment (EB, black triangles) compared to reproductive behavior (lordosis quotient) levels if estradiol benzoate (EB) was given alone (black circles). The degree of interference with estrogen-stimulated lordosis behavior was greater with a higher dose of T3 (*A*) than with a lower dose (*B*). The opposite experiment, reducing thyroid hormone levels, correspondingly led to the opposite result (*C, D*). That is, thyroidectomized animals (TX/OVX, filled circles) had better lordosis behavior responses to estradiol than did simple ovariectomized females (OVX, open circles, *C*), even if a background treatment of T3 also was given (*D*). This experiment proves the role of *endogenous* thyroid hormones in reducing the behavioral response to administered estrogen. (From Dellovade et al., 1996.)

1991; Webster et al., 1991a, b; Dahl et al., 1995; Thrun et al. 1997), high thyroid hormone levels militate against the activation of reproductive mechanisms. Thyroxine reduces estrogenic stimulation of the pituitary gene promoter. In addition, in women, thyroid abnormalities can disrupt normal passage through the menstrual cycle. In hyperthyroidism, the timing of ovulation is erratic, and menstruation becomes relatively scanty (McKenzie & Zakarija, 1995), whereas in hypothroidism possibly no ovulatory surge may occur, and women therefore tend to have irregular, anovulatory cycles with excessive menstrual bleeding (Utiger, 1995).

Synergistic and competitive relations in the surface of neural mechanisms can proceed using a variety of mechanisms (Pfaff et al., 1996; see figure 6.15). The important result is that TRs interacting with ERs can influence hypothalamic gene expression in a manner consonant with the governance of reproductive behavior. In doing so, these nuclear protein interactions render the behavior relevant to environmental circumstances, such as intolerable cold.

The principle established by this finding is that *transcription factors can interact with each other in the nuclei of hypothalamic neurons to influence behavior. These findings open up a new level of neuronal integration.* During most of the twentieth century, neurobiologists appealed to the complexity of synaptic relationships and electrophysiological mechanisms to explain integrative properties of the nervous system, but we could not explain molar behaviors. Superimposed on the anatomical-physiological levels of explanation was a second level of explanation based on the neurochemistry of neurotransmitters and neuropeptides. These new neurochemical techniques became more powerful during the last 30 years or so. Now, based on the findings reviewed here and other findings in the hormonal control of reproductive behavior, we propose a new level of neuronal integration superimposed on the first two. Interactions among transcription factors around well-recognized DNA response elements can embody the combinatorial logic required for the proper governance of instinctive behaviors. Sometimes, these interactions are competitive, and at other times they are synergistic. In any case, they have the properties expected for the biologically adaptive governance of a sophisticated molar mammalian behavior.

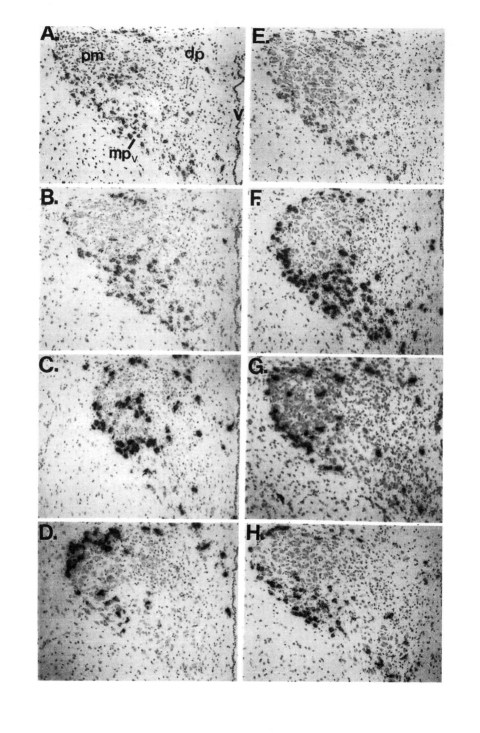

4. Gene Products Permitting Signals from
Neuron Surface to Cell Nucleus

While some of the most incisive examples of genetic influences on reproductive behavior and on the genetic components of hormone action on the brain depend on nuclear receptors that are transcription factors, it must never be forgotten that every nerve cell's responses to hormones are conditioned by inputs from the cell surface. Synaptic inputs signal stimuli from potential mates and a variety of environmental events that must be coordinated with hormonal state for the proper management of reproductive behavior.

Several experiments have been done to prove interactions between hormonal and synaptic inputs at the messenger RNA level.

Importance of Synaptic Inputs Even during the Onset of Estradiol Actions for the Induction of Enkephalin Messenger RNA and Reproductive Behavior

In 1985, Roy et al. (1985) astounded their colleagues by showing that deep anesthesia of female rats, specifically during the first application of estradiol in a hormone-priming paradigm, would block the eventual appearance of hormone-stimulated reproductive behavior. Having read that, we reflected that the enkephalin gene is remarkably sensitive to estrogen, its expression level responding very quickly, and therefore would be activated in a similar way early in the train of events after estrogenic stimulation. Therefore, that notion suggested the

Figure 7.11   (For a color reproduction of this figure, see plate 8.) Effects of estrogens with or without thyroid hormone coadministration on oxytocin gene expression in the paraventricular nucleus (PVN) of the rat hypothalamus. In situ hybridization was used to identify cells with oxytocin mRNA, and the number of grains per cell is proportional to the amount of mRNA. From sections in the PVN, representative photomicrographs of simple ovariectomized animals are shown (*A–D, left*), and sections from thyroidectomized-ovariectomized females are illustrated (*E–H, right*). Vehicle-treated females (*A, E*); estradiol-treated females (*B, F*); T3-treated females (*C, G*); and coadministration of EB and T3 (*D, H*). Also see figure 10.4 for quantitative results of this experiment. (From Dellovade et al., 1998.)

possibility that the estrogenic induction of enkephalin (or its failure in anesthetized animals) could be part of the reason for the behavioral findings of Roy et al. (1985). Indeed, enkephalin is induced very rapidly by estrogen (Romano et al., 1989b). Furthermore, messenger RNA levels for enkephalin are correlated tightly with the female rat's reproductive behavior (Lauber et al., 1990a). Moreover, enkephalin acting through δ-receptors in the forebrain or the midbrain appears to stimulate reproductive behaviors in female rats (Pfaus & Pfaff, 1992). The very nature of the opioid peptide's effects on sex behavior renders likely that enkephalins acting through δ-receptors could foster early events in reproductive behavior chains, eventually leading to reproduction, rather than simply closing the switches in a lordosis reflex loop.

Thus, we performed experiments to determine whether anesthesia could affect the induction of the enkephalin gene by estradiol parallel to the effect of anesthesia on reproductive behavior. Ovariectomized female rats either were or were not given estradiol benzoate and, in each of these two experimental groups, animals either were or were not anesthetized with pentobarbital at the time of estrogen administration (Quiñones-Jenab et al., 1996). In the absence of anesthesia, we were able to demonstrate a handsome estrogen effect on enkephalin messenger RNA in the ventromedial nucleus of the hypothalamus. However, in the presence of pentobarbital anesthesia, no significant effect on enkephalin was observed. In a control brain region, the caudate nucleus, this pattern of results did not occur. We infer that synaptic inputs arriving at the hypothalamus around the time of estrogen administration are themselves required for eventual induction of enkephalin transcription by the steroid hormone effect. These data thus provide evidence of a synergistic interaction between a hormonal input and a synaptic input.

A further possibility is that the early response by the enkephalin gene to estradiol in the skein of estradiol action itself constitutes part of the reason that, in the work of Roy et al. (1985), an eventual anesthesia effect on behavior was seen. Cellular actions of enkephalins—due to estradiol but blockable by anesthesia—near the time of estradiol administration may trigger early behavioral effects that themselves are required for the later hormone actions on lordosis behavior.

In control experiments, we determined that not simply any environmental manipulation that was effective behaviorally would also make a corresponding alteration in enkephalin gene expression (Brown et al., 1993). Axelson and Sawin (1987) at Holy Cross had reported previously that access to a locomotor activity wheel will raise animals' behavioral sensitivity to estradiol with respect to lordosis quotients. When we performed the equivalent behavioral manipulation but instead measured enkephalin messenger RNA, we did not see any specific interaction between the opportunity for locomotion and affected animals' sensitivity to estradiol as measured by enkephalin messenger RNA (Brown et al., 1993). By comparison, the effect of anesthesia (documented earlier) blocks the estrogen effect on enkephalin gene expression in a manner that seems fairly specific.

A Different Kind of Interaction: Noxious Inputs with Hormonal Inputs Determining Enkephalin Gene Expression

Because enkephalins, as opioid peptides, have been shown to be responsive to a variety of somatosensory inputs and, indeed, to participate in certain modes of analgesia and because, in parallel, we showed the sensitivity of enkephalin messenger RNA levels to estradiol and progesterone (e.g., Romano et al., 1990), a reasonable hypothesis is that these two types of influence on this particular opioid peptide gene interact (Holtzman et al., 1992, 1997). In this new experiment, the effects of estradiol and progesterone facilitating expression of the enkephalin gene in the rat VMH were replicated. However, in the presence of a continuing noxious stimulus due to subcutaneous formalin injection in one rat paw, the role of progesterone after estrogen treatment actually was reversed. Surprisingly, though in control animals with no formalin injection in the paw, progesterone *amplified* the estrogen effect, in rats injected with formalin, progesterone was associated with *fewer* grains per cell after in situ hybridization assays (Holtzman et al., 1992; unpublished data). Furthermore, these results were specific to the hypothalamus, as the same endocrine effect did not occur on enkephalin cells in the spinal cord. Here, therefore, is a different type of interaction between synaptic inputs and hormonal inputs on gene expression in hypothalamic neurons important for behavior.

***

Somatosensory and Hormonal Influences Interacting on GnRH Neurons

The *fos* gene is an early response gene wherein activation signals the response of certain types of cells to physiological challenges. Appearance of c-*fos* immunoreactivity in neurons has become a popular histochemical marker for tracking "activating" inputs to various groups of nerve cells. Cervical stimulation, for example, can lead to *fos*-identified cells in hypothalamic and limbic structures (Tetel et al., 1994). In some of these structures, such as the bed nucleus of the stria terminalis, a high percentage of *fos*-immunoreactive neurons were shown also to have ER immunoreactivity. Thus, the morphological basis for an intersection between a tactile and a hormonal stimulus was present in these and other limbic and hypothalamic cell groups.

Other investigators (Pfaus et al., 1993; Rowe & Erskine, 1993) also have found populations of neurons that respond to cervical stimulation with an increase in the hypothalamic expression of *fos*. In a new attempt to search for interactions between sensory inputs and circulating sex steroid hormone levels, we examined *fos* immunoreactivity specifically within GnRH-expressing neurons with or without estrogen–progesterone treatment and cervical stimulation (Pfaus et al., 1994). Although very few GnRH neurons coexpressed c-*fos* after steroid hormone treatment alone, cervical stimulation specifically enhanced the number of GnRH neurons that coexpress c-*fos*. Such data indicated that estrogen and progesterone can augment the responsiveness of a subset of GnRH neurons to peripheral stimulation.

Signaling from Neuron Surface Using G Proteins

Having shown that behaviorally important sensory inputs could interact with hormones in the determination of gene expression important for behavior, a seemingly legitimate inquiry is determining which signaling pathways would be used as the excitation from synaptic input traveled toward the cell nucleus. Amazingly, a tremendous portion of the list of agents that influence lordosis behavior through actions in hypothalamic neurons use the inositol phosphate signal transduction pathway (tables 7.1 and 7.2). Thus, in this particular form of

Table 7.1 Comparison of effects of neurotransmitters or neuropeptides on lordosis behavior, neuronal electrical activity, and membrane enzymes

Agonists (receptor)	Effects on			
	Lordosis behavior	Neuronal activity	Second messenger systems	
			PI system	AC system
NE (α_{1b})	↑ 75,80,81,147	↑ 147	↑ 103,185,272	
mACh (M3?)	↑ 57,58,127,235,236	↑ 140,144	↑ 73,82,100	↓ 49
5-HT (5-HT$_2$)	↑ 122,181,182,297	↑ 3,146	↑ 23,44,131,250	
LHRH	↑ 198,239,240,247,248	~ 207,210	↑ 34,249	↑ 7,152,200,265
SP (NK 1?)	↑ 63	↑ 207	↑ 167,289	
OT	↑ 254	↑ 137,141	↑ 8,92,168,169,244	
PRL	↑ 109	_ 207,209, ↑ 34	↑ 5,74	
TRH	↑ ★, _ 109,239,240	↑ 144	↑ 133,171,172,230	
GABA$_A$	↑ 176,49,177	↓ 140,205,206	↑ 47,242	
5-HT (5-HT$_{1A}$)	↓ 161,163	↓ 140,146	↓ 155	↓ 56,115,303
DA (D$_2$)	↓ 98	↓ 140,287	↓ 155,165,197	↓ 48,52
NPY	↓ 38,125	↓ 6,43		↓ 88,126
β-End (μ)	↓ 260,263,293	↓ 68		↓ 37
CRF	↓ 262	↑ 69,302, ↓ 259		↑ 4,148
αMSH	↓ 226			↓ 2
ACTH	↓ 28,53	_ 209	↓ 155	↓ 274
CCK	↓ 10,17	↑ 142,257	↑ 255	↑ 159
EAAs (NMDA,KA)	↓ 136,175	↑ 136	↓ 11,93,124,155,201,252	↓ 121
AVP	↑ 28,72 ↓ 30,266	↑ 137,141	↑ 18	↓ 178,193

↑, stimulatory; ↓, inhibitory; −, no effect; ~, modulatory; PI, phosphatidyl inositol; AC, adenylate cyclase; NE, norepinephrine (α_{1b} receptors); mACh, muscarinic acetylcholine receptors; 5-HT, serotonin; SP, substance P; OT, oxytocin; PRL, prolactin; TRM, TSM releasing hormone; DA, dopamine; NPY, neuropeptide Y; β-End, β-endorphin (μ receptors); CRF, corticotropin releasing factor; αMSM, α-melanocyte stimulating hormone; CCK, cholecystekinin; EAAs, excitatory amino acids; AVP, arginine vaspressin. See text for other abbreviations.

Notes: Superscript numbers are references: see Kow et al. (1994).
★Kow & Pfaff, unpublished.
Source: Kow et al. (1994).

Table 7.2 Effects of estrogens on the phosphoinositide second-messenger system

Items examined	Effects	Preparations	Estrogen	Treatment		References
				Conc./dose	Duration	
G proteins (G_o, G_{i3})	Specific changes	Rat pituitary	E2	10 μg/rat/day	> 5 days	(21)
G proteins ($G_i2\alpha$, $G_i3\alpha$)	Selective changes	Rat myometrium	E2	Endogenous		(273)
GTPase	↑	Rat anterior pituitary homogenates	E2	10^{-7} M	< 5 min	(229)
Incorporation of [3H]myoinositol	↑	Immature mouse uterus	DES	5 μg/kg, IP	< 60 min	(118)
Incorporation of [3H]myoinositol	↑	Ewe uterine tissue	EB	750 μg/ewe/day × 2	24 hr	(114)
Incorporation [3H]myoinositol	↑	Mouse uterine tissue	DES	5 μg/kg	1–3 hr	(99)
Incorporation [3H]myoinositol	↑	MCF-7 human breast cancer cells	E2	10^{-9} M	4–24 hr	(78)
PLC activity	↑ then ↓	MCF-7 cells or homogenates	E2, but not α-E2 or P_4	10^{-12}–10^{-6} M	↑, 5 sec ↓, 5 min	(97)
PLCα	Induced	Rat VMN	E2	100% in capsule	14 hr	(190, 191)
PLC activity	↑	MCF-7 cells	E2	10^{-12} M	24 hr	(89)
PLC activity	↑	MCF-7 cells	E2	10^{-12}–10^{-10} M	4 days	(275)
Inositol phosphates	↑	Immature mouse uterus	DES	5 μg/kg, IP	< 60 min	(118)

PKC activity	↑ or ↓	Rat brain soluble extract	DPEs	2–200 μ M	3.5 min	(15)
PKC	Translocated	Rat mammary gland tumors and uterine tissue	E2	10 μg/rat, IP	10–15 min	(258)
PKC activity	↑	Membrane of estrogen-target tissue	E2	5×10^{-9} M	20 min	(196)
PKC activity	↑	Rat pituitary in vivo and in vitro	E2, but not α-E2	Capsule or 10^{-9} M	24 hr	(65)
PKC activity	↑	Rat luteal fraction	E2	100% in capsule	72 hr	(269)
PDBu-induced LH release	↑	Rat ovariectomized	E2	100% in capsule	4–5 days	(278)
NE-induced PI hydrolysis	↑	Rat cerebral cortical slices	EB	2 or 10 μg/rat, SC	> 24 hr	(79)
NE (α$_1$)-evoked PI hydrolysis	↑	Rabbit uterine tissue	EB	50 μg/kg/day × 4	4 days	(237)
OT-evoked PI hydrolysis	↑	Ewe uterine tissue	EB	750 μg/ewe/day × 2	24 hr	(114)
GnRH-evoked PI hydrolysis	↑	Rat granulosa cells	E2, but not P$_4$	10^{-7} M	30 min and 48 hr	(119)

DES, diethylstilbestrol; DPEs, 1,1-diphenylethylene derivates; E2,17β-estradiol; α-E2, 17α-estradiol; EB,17β-estradiol benzoate; IP, intraperitoneal injection; P$_4$, progesterone; PDBu, phorbol 12,13-dibutyrate; SC, subcutaneous injection; G proteins; guanine diphosphate and triphosphate binding proteins; PLC, phospholipase C; PKC, protein kinase C. See also table 7.1 and text.

For references, see Kow et al. (1994).

Source: Kow et al. (1994).

neural plasticity—the change from an unreceptive animal to an animal that would perform a reproductive behavior response—the key pathway seems not to be routed through cyclic AMP or protein kinase A but instead through phospholipase C, inositol phosphate, and protein kinase C (Kow et al., 1994). Targeting this pathway allowed us, in turn, to ask the more detailed question of whether particular G proteins were involved and, if so, *which* proteins were involved (figure 7.12). A long series of electrophysiological, Western blot, reverse transcriptase–polymerase chain reaction, and antisense DNA experiments (Kow et al., 1997a,b) led to the conclusion that signaling through Gq (α_{11}) must be essential for the signaling of adrenergic transmitters on VMH neurons (Kow & Pfaff, 1997b). As norepinephrine is released at synaptic terminals in the VMH, it acts through α_{1a} and α_{1b} receptors to activate Gq α_{11} among the panoply of G proteins. Gq α_{11}, acting in turn through phospholipase C isoform β_1, allows the production of diacylglycerol, which in turn activates protein kinase C (figures 7.13 and 7.14). Previously, we showed that the activation of protein kinase C is associated with increased VMH neuronal activity, in turn required for the activation of lordosis behavior (Kow et al., 1994, 1997). In some detail, therefore, a signal transduction pathway participating in the interaction between synaptic inputs and hormonal inputs to hypothalamic neurons has been unraveled.

B. INFLUENCES OF GENES ON BEHAVIOR

Using gene knockout animals and antisense DNA technology, it has been possible to establish both direct and indirect effects of genes on female reproductive behavior and other sexually differentiated behaviors (see later). Of course, not all effects of estrogens or progestins on the nervous system are genomic (Moss et al., 1997). However, because RNA and protein synthesis inhibitors, gene knockouts, and antisense DNA microinjections in the brain are so highly effective in blocking the effects of estrogens and progestins on reproductive behavior, the assumption is that genomic mechanisms are essential for regulating this behavior and carry the main causal load.

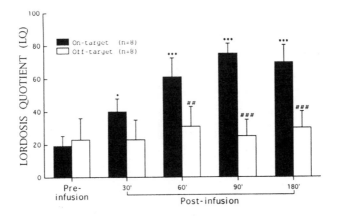

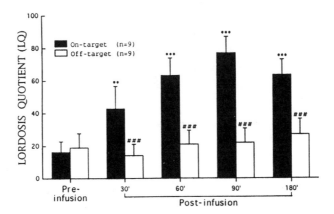

Figure 7.12   (*Top*) Infusion of (TPA) to activate protein kinase C directly into the ventro-medial nucleus of the hypothalamus (black bars) significantly facilitated lordosis behavior. Attempts at medial hypothalamic infusions that were off-target had no significant effect. (*Bottom*) Infusion of TPA to activate protein kinase C into the midbrain central gray facilitated lordosis behavior, whereas attempted infusions that were off-target had no significant effect. (From Kow et al., 1994.)

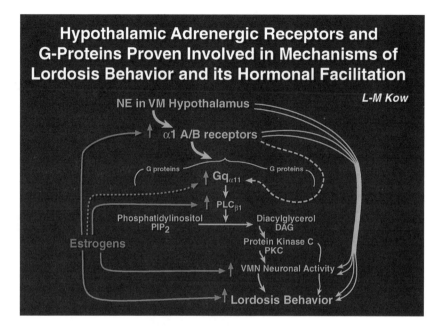

Figure 7.13 (For a color reproduction of their figure, see plate 9.) A series of electrophysiological and pharmacological experiments has shown how hypothalamic adrenergic receptors and specific G proteins are involved in mechanisms of lordosis behavior and its hormonal facilitation. Results, primarily from the work of Kow and his colleagues, involving adrenergic receptors, Gqα11 and protein kinase C are shown in green. Five sites of estrogenic facilitation are shown in red.

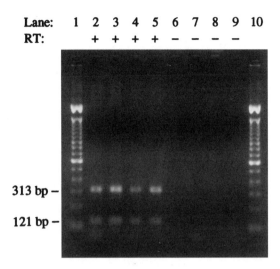

Figure 7.14   The G proteins implicated in behaviorally relevant signal transduction in lordosis mechanisms are expressed in ventromedial hypothalamus. The reverse transcriptase–polymerase chain rection (RT-PCR) technique was used. Lanes 1 and 10 are molecular weight ladders, with the expected size products for G-α11 (121 bp) and G-αq (313 bp) indicated. Lanes 2 to 5 had samples treated with RT, whereas lanes 6 to 9 were controls without RT. Lanes 2 and 6 are samples from ventromedial hypothalamus; lanes 3 and 7, cerebral cortex; 4 and 8, kidney; and 5 and 9, caudate-putamen (Kow et al., 1997). Note also that in related experiments intra-VMH (but not intrathalamic) infusion of antisense DNA against mRNA for G-α11 (but not control substances) blocked adrenergic neurotransmitter α_1-agonist induced lordosis facilitation (Kow et al., 1996).

PRINCIPLES OF GENE BEHAVIOR RELATIONS

Effects of genes on mammalian behaviors can be either direct or indirect (table 7.3), even for simple hormone-stimulated reproductive behaviors (Ogawa et al., 1996a).

1. DIRECT EFFECTS

Relatively direct effects of genes on mammalian social behavior during adulthood are shown clearly by estrogens and progestins working through their cognate nuclear ERs and progestin receptors to control female reproductive behaviors. Female mice with the classical ER gene knocked out (ERKO) simply do not show estrogen-dependent reproductive behavior (table 7.4). Even with their ovarian hormones circulating, ERKO female mice are so aggressive that they not only refuse to perform reproductive behavior but attack the male (Ogawa et al., 1996b). This genetic result with sex behavior follows readily from the fact that ER binding is strong in brain regions known to control female reproductive behavior (Pfaff, 1968; Pfaff & Keiner, 1973) and from stud-

Table 7.3 Scheme charting all possible gene-behavior causal routes, *not* mutually exclusive★

	Through development		During adulthood	
Locus	Lethal	Not lethal	Sensorimotor	Integrative
Direct on brain	Indirect	Indirect	Direct	Direct
Action outside brain	Indirect	Indirect	Indirect	Indirect

★Further subdivisions will be necessary as data proliferate.
Note: Considering adult behavior, all actions of genes on development, including mutations of hormone receptors and alterations of enzymes for steroid hormone synthesis and metabolism, would be considered *indirect*. *Direct* effects would include genes expressed in the brain in adulthood that are necessary for a particular behavior, including genes for hormone receptors and hormone metabolism.
Source: Adapted from Ogawa et al., 1996a.

Table 7.4 Complete loss of lordosis behavior due to ER gene deletion

	Incidence of female reproductive behavior	Incidence of female-female aggression
Wild type	Normal	2/21 mice
Estrogen receptor knockout	None	10/25 mice★

★Aggression exhibited by estrogen receptor knockout females mainly offensive attacks typical of intermale aggression.
Source: Based on data from Ogawa et al., 1996b.

ies that used ER blockers (Etgen, 1979; Luttge, 1976; Morin et al., 1976; Pfaff et al., 1994; Roy & Wade, 1977; Walker & Feder, 1977a,b).

Likewise, PR gene expression is required for progestin effects on female reproductive behavior. Antisense DNA directed against PR messenger RNA microinjected into the VMH significantly reduces female reproductive behavior (figure 7.15; Ogawa, 1994) and, even more impressively, reduced progestin-dependent courtship behaviors by 80%, down to 20% of control levels (Ogawa et al., 1994). Indeed, progestin receptor induction is correlated perfectly with the onset of female rat reproductive behavior (Parsons et al., 1980, 1982a,b; Pleim et al., 1989; Rubin & Barfield, 1983), and progestin receptor blockers, such as RU486 (Brown & Blaustein, 1984; Etgen & Barfield, 1986; Vathy et al., 1987), partially block the effects of progesterone on female reproductive behavior. Progesterone acting through PR has behaviorally important synthetic consequences, as shown by the blocking action of protein synthesis inhibitor anisomycin (Glaser & Barfield, 1984). In perfect accord with all these data, Lydon et al. (1995) found that PR gene knockout female mice demonstrated no effect of progesterone on female mouse lordosis behavior. Even in PR knockout mice that were studied in our laboratory and in which estrogen-stimulated lordosis was apparent, the progesterone effect on female reproductive behavior was eliminated (table 7.5; Ogawa et al., 1998).

As regards *assay conditions,* even slight increases in the complexity of the behavior analyzed can lead to corresponding complexity of assay and interpretation. Consider maternal behavior in rats (Fahrbach et al., 1986). In support of

(A) Lordosis Quotient

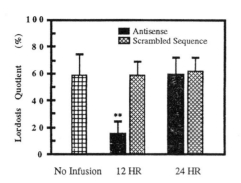

(B) Lordosis Reflex Intensity

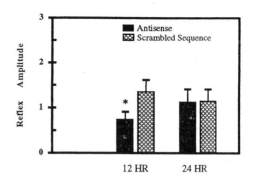

(C) Proceptive Behavior

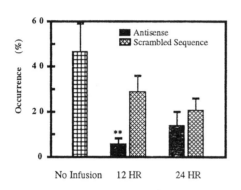

(D) Rejection Behavior

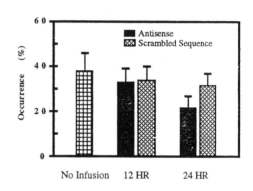

(E) Vocalization

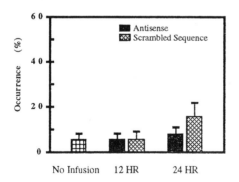

Table 7.5   Reproductive behavior of progesterone receptor knockout females

	Estrogenic facilitation of lordosis?	Progesterone magnification of estrogen effect?
Wild type	Yes	Yes
Progesterone receptor knockout	Yes	No

maternal behavior, estrogen administration can increase the amount of oxytocin messenger RNA in a small subset of oxytocinergic neurons in the paraventricular nucleus of the hypothalamus (Chung et al., unpublished data; Dellovade et al., in press) and also can turn on the gene for the oxytocin receptor in the brain (Bale & Dorsa, 1995; Quiñones-Jenab et al., 1997). These dependencies of oxytocin function and a consideration of the peripheral roles of oxytocin in giving birth and in lactation render eminently sensible that oxytocin should be able to stimulate maternal behavior. Yet the relationship of the gene products, oxytocin and its receptor, to maternal behavior can be demonstrated only under specific assay conditions. If the female rat is totally unstressed or if she is highly stressed, showing an oxytocin effect on maternal behavior is difficult. In the intermediate case, if she has received mild stress, the oxytocin effect is strong and statistically significant (Fahrbach et al., 1986). In fact, a mechanism for the Fahrbach effect recently may have been discovered in the anxiolytic action of

Figure 7.15   Temporary interference with expression of a specific gene in hypothalamic neurons can reduce certain sociosexual behaviors. (*A*) Antisense DNA directed against progesterone receptor mRNA significantly reduced the frequency of lordosis behavior in female rats. It then recovered, showing that the experimental manipulation had not simply damaged the ventromedial hypothalamic neurons involved. (*B*) Likewise, the amplitude of lordosis responses, when they occurred, also were reduced. (*C*) Courtship behaviors ("proceptive behaviors") of female rats are known to depend especially heavily on progesterone. They were reduced greatly (by 80%) after PR antisense DNA microinjection amidst medial hypothalamic neurons. Then they recovered. (*D, E*). Neither rejection behaviors nor vocalizations were affected, indicating behavioral specificity of the antisense DNA effect. (From Ogawa et al., 1994.)

centrally administered oxytocin (Windle et al., 1997). The relevant principle is that *demonstration of the relationship between a specific gene and a particular mammalian behavior depends exquisitely on the precise conditions of assay.*

2. INDIRECT EFFECTS

Some of the best examples of indirect effects of genes on behavior derive from demonstrations of sex differences. On the Y chromosome, expression of SRY allows development of testes at the expense of ovaries. The resulting effects of testicular hormones on the brain provide a rich array of examples clearly relating genes to behavior.

In turn, the configuration of data gathered in this and other laboratories demonstrates that the exact nature of these genetic effects on behavior depends on exactly where and exactly when the gene is expressed and even the gender of the animal in which it is expressed. Take the ER in the genetic female. Use of antisense DNA against the ER messenger RNA microinjected into the neonatal hypothalamus of female rats can *prevent* the masculinization of brain and behavior produced by an experimental testosterone injection in these neonatal female rats (McCarthy et al., 1993). In dramatic contrast, permanent interruption of the ER gene in tissues throughout the body, as achieved in the ERKO mouse, yields a female mouse that is *more masculinized;* these animals behave less like genetic females and are treated as males (table 7.6). A comparison of these two results on the nature of the ER gene product and its contribution to masculinization of the brain (figure 7.16) yields the following principle: *The effect of a gene on a specific behavior depends on exactly where and exactly when that gene is expressed.*

Another principle of gene actions on behavior (see figure 7.16) derives from comparing the effect of the ERKO in the female to that in the genetic male. Surprisingly, ERKO males show virtually no intromissions or ejaculations, they lack male typical aggressive behavior, and their emotionality in an open field is more like that of a female (table 7.7). Overall, these ERKO males show a strong trend toward a more feminine type of behavioral profile. A comparison of this result to the opposite result in genetic females yields the follow-

Table 7.6 Behavioral masculinization of female mice as a result of estrogen receptor gene knockout

Alterations in ERKO females	
Maternal behavior (including infanticide)	Reduced
Aggressive behavior	
Toward females	Increased
Toward males	Increased
Female reproductive behavior	Abolished

Source: From Ogawa et al., 1996b.

ing principle: *The effect of a gene on the development of behavior can depend on the gender of the animal in which that gene is expressed.*

In summary, it is amazing that the same gene for the nuclear hormone receptor for estradiol is absolutely necessary both for a full pattern of masculine behavior in the genetic male and for a full pattern of feminine behavior in the genetic female. Thus, even though *masculization* and *feminization* typically are considered to be names for opposite ends of a continuum in reproductive biology, normal expression of the gene for the ER is necessary for both types of behavior.

Kallmann's Syndrome in Humans

A human syndrome provides an example of how subtle and indirect relationships between genes and behavior can be. Kallmann's syndrome—hypogonadotropic hypogonadism—afflicts men with an obvious behavioral change: the absence of libido as part of a lack of interest in the opposite sex. Causation of X-linked Kallmann's syndrome now is understood in light of our surprising finding that GnRH neurons are not born as expected near ventricular surfaces in the brain but instead are born in the olfactory epithelium (Schwanzel-Fukuda & Pfaff, 1989, 1992). GnRH neurons, having been born in the developing olfactory sensory surface, undertake to migrate up the nose and along the bottom of the brain,

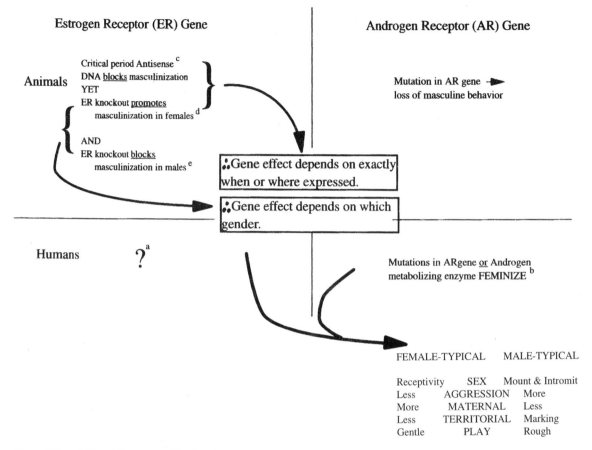

(A) PARTICIPATION OF GENES FOR NUCLEAR RECEPTORS IN SEXUALLY DIFFERENTIATED BEHAVIORS IN MAMMALS

Estrogen Receptor (ER) Gene

Androgen Receptor (AR) Gene

Animals

Critical period Antisense [c]
DNA <u>blocks</u> masculinization
YET
ER knockout <u>promotes</u>
masculinization in females [d]

AND
ER knockout <u>blocks</u>
masculinization in males [e]

Mutation in AR gene →
loss of masculine behavior

∴Gene effect depends on exactly when or where expressed.

∴Gene effect depends on which gender.

Humans   ? [a]

Mutations in ARgene <u>or</u> Androgen metabolizing enzyme FEMINIZE [b]

	FEMALE-TYPICAL		MALE-TYPICAL
Receptivity	SEX	Mount & Intromit
Less	AGGRESSION	More
More	MATERNAL	Less
Less	TERRITORIAL	Marking
Gentle	PLAY	Rough

Figure 7.16 (*A*) Dual illustration of the facts that certain sociosexual behaviors clearly depend on specific genes, but also that these dependencies can be so complex that systematic understanding rests upon the elucidation of the underlying physiology. (*Top,* ER) Antisense DNA application causing an interruption of ER gene function (McCarthy et al., 1993) that is limited in time and space gives a much different behavioral result than that (Ogawa et al., 1996b) after estrogen receptor gene knockout (ERKO), which applies throughout the body for the entire life of the organism. (*Bottom,* ER) In turn, behavioral results with ERKO males (Ogawa et al., 1997) are not the same as those with ERKO females (Ogawa et al., 1996b). The behavioral effect of a gene can depend on the gender of the organism in which it is expressed. [a]One reported case, a male "with low libido"; [b]More detail in text; [c]McCarthy et al., 1993; [d]Ogawa et al., 1996; [e]Ogawa et al., 1997. (*B*) Participation of genes for nuclear receptors in brain mechanisms for reproductive behaviors in adult experimental animals. The simplest causal relationships are illustrated here. For clarity, roles of E and P in males and AR in females are left out. References for the three major segments are as follows: *Estrogen receptor (ER):* [a]Pfaff, 1968; Pfaff and Keiner, 1973; [b]Lauber et al., 1991; Simerly et al., 1992; [c]Blaustein et al., [d]Gorski et al.,; [e]Ogawa, 1996. *Progesterone receptor (PR):* [a]MacLusky and McEwen, 1978; Parsons et al., 1980, 1982; Sar and Stumpf; Blaustein; [b]Romano, 1989; [c]Blaustein; [d]Romano, 1989; Lauber, 1991; [e]Vathy and Brown; [f]Ogawa et al., 1994; Mani et al., 1997; Pollio and Maggi, 1994; [g]Lydon et al., 1995; Ogawa et al., 1998. *Androgen receptor (AR):* [a]McEwen et al., 1970; Sar & Stumpf; Whalen & Clemens; [b]Simerly et al., 1990; [c]Sodersten et al., 1985; [d]Meisel & Sachs, 1994; [e]Ohno et al., 1971; Olsen et al., 1982.

(B)

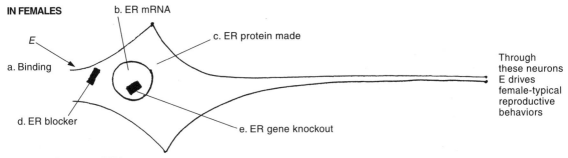

IN FEMALES

b. ER mRNA

E

c. ER protein made

a. Binding

d. ER blocker

e. ER gene knockout

Through these neurons E drives female-typical reproductive behaviors

Estrogen Receptor (ER)
a. ER binding present in behavior-controlling nerve cell groups.
b. ER mRNA present in behavior-controlling nerve cell groups.
c. ER immuno-reactive protein present in behavior-controlling nerve cell groups.

d. ER receptor blocker reduces lordosis.
e. ER gene knockout abolishes lordosis.

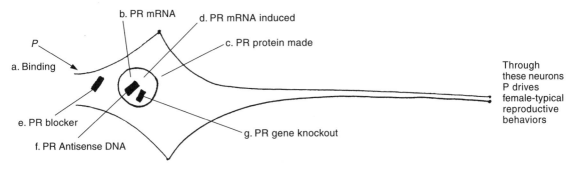

b. PR mRNA   d. PR mRNA induced

P

c. PR protein made

a. Binding

e. PR blocker

f. PR Antisense DNA

g. PR gene knockout

Through these neurons P drives female-typical reproductive behaviors

Progesterone Receptor (PR)
a. PR binding present in behavior-controlling nerve cell groups.
b. PR mRNA present in behavior-controlling nerve cell groups.
c. PR immuno-reactive protein present in behavior-controlling nerve cell groups.
d. PR mRNA induced by E parallel to behavior.

e. PR receptor blocker reduces lordosis.
f. PR Antisense DNA greatly reduces lordosis and courtship behaviors.
g. PR gene knockout blocks P-facilitated lordosis (more detail in Chapter 7).

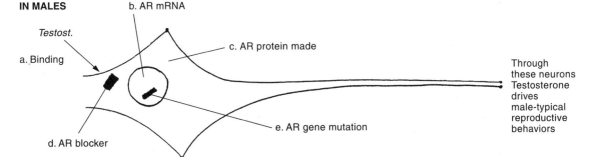

IN MALES

b. AR mRNA

Testost.

c. AR protein made

a. Binding

d. AR blocker

e. AR gene mutation

Through these neurons Testosterone drives male-typical reproductive behaviors

Androgen Receptor (AR)
a. AR binding present in behavior-controlling nerve cell groups.
b. AR mRNA present in behavior-controlling nerve cell groups.
c. AR immuno-reactive protein present in behavior-controlling nerve cell groups.

d. AR receptor blocker reduces mating.
e. AR gene mutation abolishes mating.

Table 7.7   Behavioral feminization of male mice as a result of estrogen receptorgene knockout

Alterations in ERKO males	
Male-specific intromissions and ejaculations	Less rare
Aggression (offensive attacks)	Less rare
Open-field (emotional) responses	Feminized

entering the brain near their final functional place in the preoptic area and anterior hypothalamus.

X-linked Kallmann's syndrome, caused by genetic damage at Xp-22.3, is correlated with a failure of migration of GnRH neurons (Schwanzel-Fukuda et al., 1989b). These GnRH neurons were born normally but, after migrating up the nose, they were dammed up in the top of the olfactory apparatus and never reached the brain. In turn, this neuronal migration disorder is rationalized by the fact that damage at Xp-22.3 disrupts a specific gene (Franco et al., 1991; Legouis et al., 1991), the damage of which causes X-linked Kallmann's syndrom. This gene codes for a cell surface protein present during migration of GnRH neurons into the brain (Dellovade et al., unpublished data; figure 7.17).

Putting these and closely related facts in a very logical order leads to a clear example of the complex participation by an individual gene in a human social behavior through its actions during development: That is, in males suffering from X-linked Kallmann's syndrome, behavioral libido is reduced *because* of low testosterone levels, which occurred in turn *because* of reduced gonadotropins (luteinizing hormone and follicle-stimulating hormone), which in turn are low *because* no GnRH arrives from the brain to enter the pituitary, *because* no GnRH neurons are found in the brain, *because* of a failure of GnRH neuronal migration, *because* of the absence of the cell surface protein produced by a gene at Xp-22.3.

The principle: *It is possible to demonstrate a genetic influence on a crucial human social behavior, but the data also illustrate the complicated and indirect nature of such an effect.*

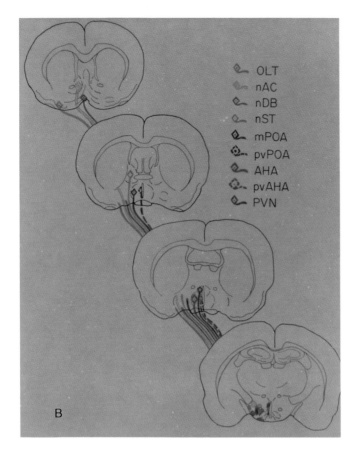

OLT
nAC
nDB
nST
mPOA
pvPOA
AHA
pvAHA
PVN

B

Plate 1 (figure 5.11)

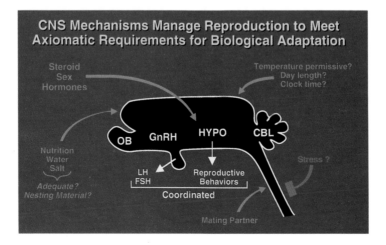

CNS Mechanisms Manage Reproduction to Meet Axiomatic Requirements for Biological Adaptation

Steroid Sex Hormones

Temperature permissive? Day length? Clock time?

Nutrition Water Salt

OB GnRH HYPO CBL

Stress ?

Adequate? Nesting Material?

LH FSH

Reproductive Behaviors

Coordinated

Mating Partner

Plate 2 (figure 6.13)

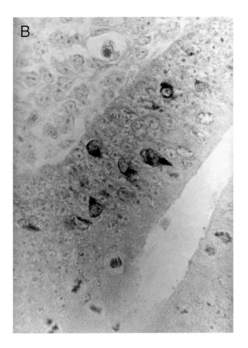

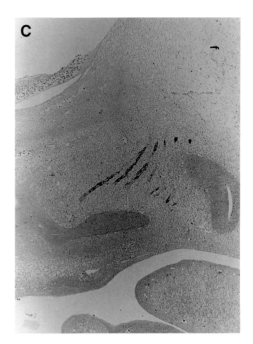

Plate 3 (figure 6.17)

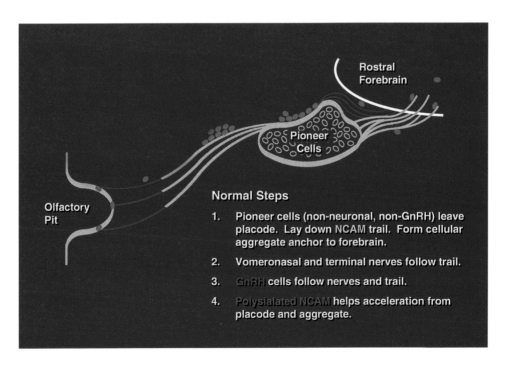

Rostral
Forebrain

Pioneer
Cells

Olfactory
Pit

Normal Steps

1. Pioneer cells (non-neuronal, non-GnRH) leave placode. Lay down NCAM trail. Form cellular aggregate anchor to forebrain.

2. Vomeronasal and terminal nerves follow trail.

3. GnRH cells follow nerves and trail.

4. Polysialated NCAM helps acceleration from placode and aggregate.

Plate 4 (figure 6.18)

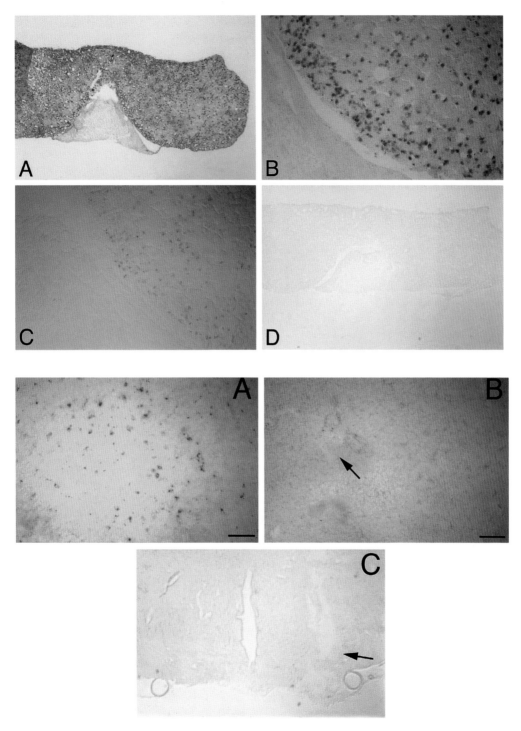

Plate 5 (figure 7.2)

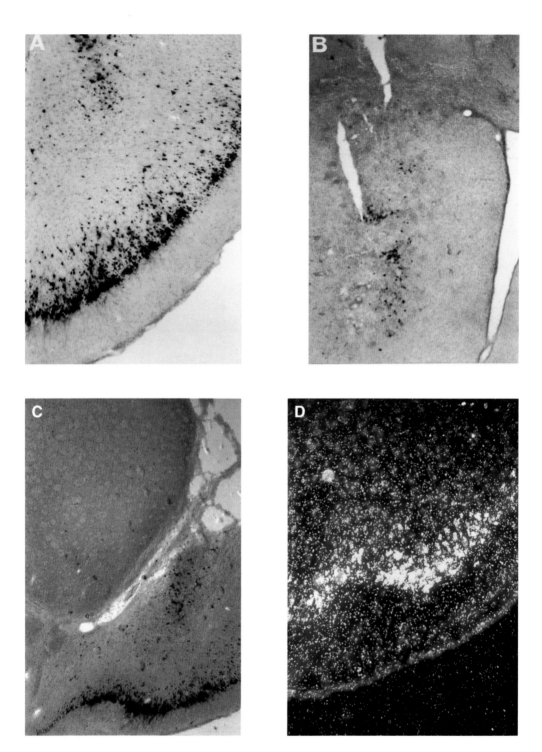

Plate 6 (figure 7.4)

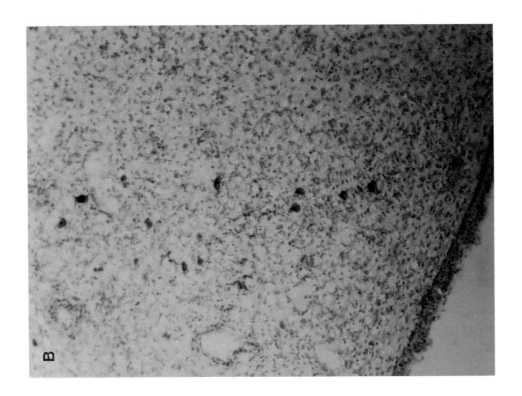

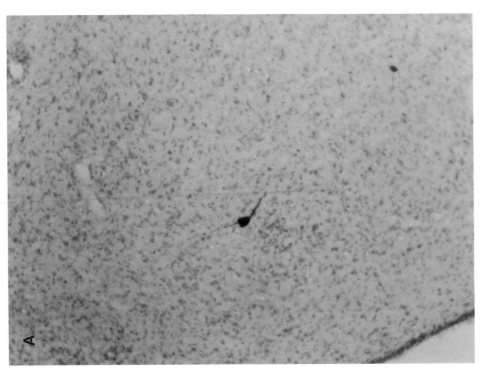

Plate 7 (figure 7.5)

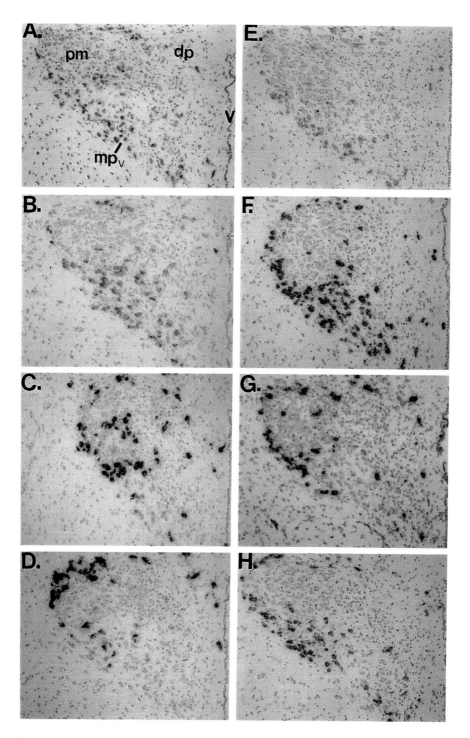

Plate 8 (figure 7.11)

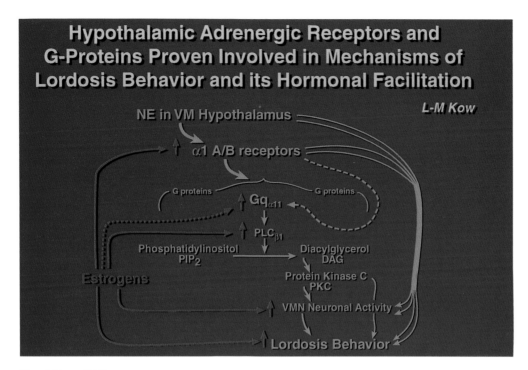

Plate 9 (figure 7.13)

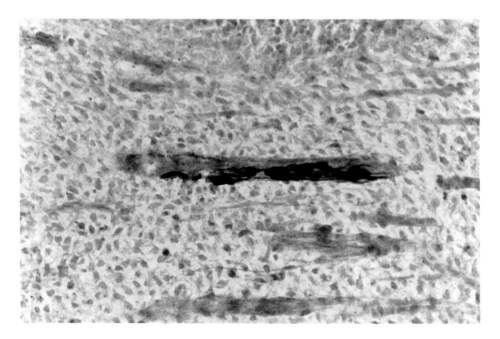

Plate 10 (figure 7. 17)

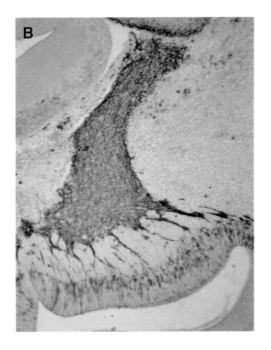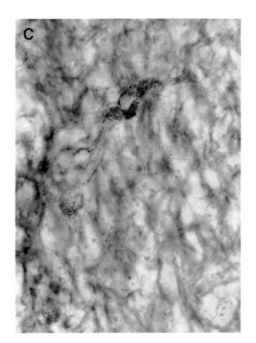

Plate 11 (figure 8.5)

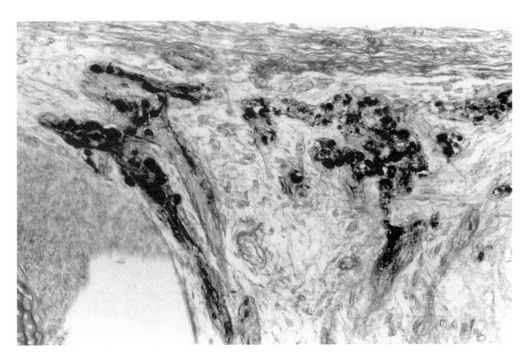

Plate 12 (figure 8.6)

Plate 1 (figure 5.11)   Efferents from the basal forebrain and anterior hypothalamus follow more orderly trajectories than had been anticipated. Axons descending from the olfactory tubercle (OLT), nucleus accumbens (NAC), nuclei of the diagonal band of Broca (NDB), nucleus of the stria terminalis (NST), medial preoptic area (MPOA), periventricular POA (PVPOA), anterior hypothalamic area (AHA), periventricular anterior hypothalamic area (PVAHA), and periventricular nucleus (PVN), have trajectories that approximate "laminar flow" (first published in Pfaff & Conrad, 1978).

Plate 2 (figure 6.13)   Because of the high biological cost of reproduction to females, the brain must manage reproductive physiology and behavior in a manner that obeys obvious biological requirements. Several environmental factors (in green) must be present within defined ranges, and stress (in red) must be minimized or it will block reproduction. As a result of neural activity in gonadotropin-releasing hormone (GnRH) neurons and in other hypothalamic (HYPO) cells, release of gonadotropins—luteinizing hormone, follicle-stimulating hormone (LH and FSH)—from the pituitary is beautifully coordinated with female reproductive behavior. We have figured out the circuitry by which steroid sex hormones in the female potentiate the behavioral effects of stimuli from the male mating partner (in green). Now we are working on how other environmental factors modulate this system. (OB, olfactory bulb; CBL, cerebellum.)

Plate 3 (figure 6.17)   (B) At high magnification, immunocytochemically stained GnRH neurons in the olfactory placode of the embryonic mouse. GnRH-expressing neurons were recognized using the antibody LR1. (C) A photomicrograph taken at lower magnification than in B and at a slightly later stage of development, showing "trains" of GnRH neurons migrating across the olfactory apparatus from the olfactory placode (near the bottom) toward the basal forebrain (f, near the top). GnRH neurons tend to migrate in clusters. (From Schwanzel-Fukuda & Pfaff, 1989.)

Plate 4 (figure 6.18)   Schematic summary of steps involved in the migration of newly born gonadotropin-releasing hormone neurons (red ovals) from the olfactory pit into the developing basal forebrain. This migration, established by the discovery of Schwanzel-Fukuda and Pfaff (1989), occurs in all vertebrates studied and is essential for the development of neural controls over reproduction. Participation by neural cell adhesion molecule (NCAM) is shown using color coding. Additional reading includes papers on NCAM and on human brain development (Schwanzel-Fukuda et al., 1992, 1994, 1996).

Plate 5 (figure 7.2)   Use of neurotropic viral vectors (herpes "amplicon") for in vivo promoter analysis. Here we ask, *in the context of normal pituitary nuclear proteins (top, A–D) or normal hypothalamic nuclear proteins (bottom)*, two questions: First, can a selected portion of the progesterone receptor promote drive transcription of a reporter gene (β-galactosidase) in appropriate pituitary or hypothalamic cells, respectively? Second, can estradiol regulate transcription of the reporter gene through the progesterone receptor promoter in those cells? (*Top, A*) Low-power photomicrograph of the rat pituitary taken from an estrogen-treated female. Note the widespread and dense expression of β-galactosidase in the anterior pituitary. As a built-in anatomical control, the posterior pituitary shows no expression of the reporter gene under this promoter. (*Top, B*) High-power photomicrograph from an estrogen-treated anterior pituitary. Dense cellular expression of the reporter gene stimulated by estrogen action through the progesterone receptor promoter is evident. (*Top, C*) In the control, vehicle-treated female rat anterior pituitary, only weak reporter gene expression is seen. (*Top, D*) As an additional viral control, when only the helper virus (without the viral vector) was injected into the sella turcica, no cells are stained. (From Scott et al., unpublished data. Molecular Brain Research, submitted, 1999). (*Bottom, A*) Ventromedial hypothalamic neurons showed significant levels of reporter gene expression stimulated by estrogen working through the progesterone receptor promoter. Every blue-green cell body seen here indicates robust progesterone receptor activity in hypothalamic neurons sampled from an estrogen-treated rat. The cells demonstrating estrogen-stimulated progesterone receptor promoter activity include the very neurons through which estrogen acts to turn on the progesterone receptor itself and lordosis behavior. (*Bottom, B*) In a control, ovariectomized female rat, hardly any reporter gene–expressing cells were seen in the medial hypothalamus, even near the viral vector injection site (arrow). (*Bottom, C*) When hypothalamic tissue was injected with the control helper virus only (no viral vector included), no staining was seen. (From Scott et al., 1998.)

Plate 6 (figure 7.4)   First use of a viral vector for in vivo promoter analysis in the central nervous system revealed region-specific and cell-specific gene expression (data from Kaplitt et al., 1994). Dr. Michael J. Kaplitt prepared a herpes simplex "amplicon" viral vector, in which 2,700 bases of the rat enkephalin promoter were placed upstream of the bacterial lacZ gene, to drive expression of that reporter gene. Thus, effective transcription through that promoter would yield blue-green nerve cells as against a violet counterstain. This viral vector was microinjected into selected regions of the rat central nervous system. Positive expression, denoted by the blue-green cells, matched endogenous enkephalin expression and is illustrated in the piriform cortex (A) and in the caudate nucleus (B). Control microinjections into regions that do not express enkephalin endogenously did not yield these collections of blue-green cells. Further, fidelity of viral vector–mediated gene expression with respect to the endogenous enkephalin gene's expression was illustrated by the excellent match between the β-galactosidase pattern in the piriform cortex (C) and the pattern shown after in situ hybridization for endogenous enkephalin messenger RNA (D).

Plate 7 (figure 7.5)   Use of a neurotropic viral vector (as described in figure 7.4) to demonstrate estrogenic regulation of the enkephalin promoter in medial hypothalamic neurons. Yin and Kaplitt prepared a herpes simplex "amplicon" viral vector in which 2,700 bases of the rat enkephalin promoter were used to drive a β-galactosidase reporter gene. This they microinjected among ventromedial hypothalamic neurons in ovariectomized female rats that then were given either vehicle control (A) or were given an injection subcutaneously with estradiol benzoate (B). Estrogen treatment clearly increased transcription through the enkephalin promoter, yielding a larger number of blue-green stained cell bodies (Yin et al., 1994, Endocrine Society Abstract and unpublished data). This finding fits with previous results (see text). These data also illustrate the first use in the CNS of a viral vector to demonstrate physiological regulation of a gene promoter.

Plate 8 (figure 7.11)   Effects of estrogens with or without thyroid hormone coadministration on oxytocin gene expression in the paraventricular nucleus (PVN) of the rat hypothalamus. In situ hybridization was used to identify cells with oxytocin mRNA, and the number of grains per cell is proportional to the amount of mRNA. From sections in the PVN, representative photomicrographs of simple ovariectomized animals are shown (A–D, left), and sections from thyroidectomized-ovariectomized females are illustrated (E–H, right). Vehicle-treated females (A, E); estradiol-treated females (B, F); T3-treated females (C, G); and coadministration of EB and T3 (D, H). Also see figure 10.4 for quantitative results of this experiment. (From Dellovade et al., 1998.)

Plate 9 (figure 7.13)   A series of electrophysiological and pharmacological experiments has shown how hypothalamic adrenergic receptors and specific G proteins are involved in mechanisms of lordosis behavior and its hormonal facilitation. Results, primarily from the work of Kow and his colleagues, involving adrenergic receptors, $Gq\alpha_{11}$ and protein kinase C are shown in green. Five sites of estrogenic facilitation are shown in red.

Plate 10 (figure 7.17)   A GnRH neuron migrating up the nasal septum toward the brain during fetal development surrounded by Anosmin I immunoreactivity. (From Dellovade et al., in press.)

Plate 11 (figure 8.5)   (*B*) Low-power photomicrograph corresponding to section 87. Even at low magnification, some of the red-brown-stained GnRH neurons are visible migrating from the olfactory pit (aperture at bottom) to the basal forebrain (*top*). (*C*) At higher magnification, red-brown-stained GnRH neurons, recognized immunocytochemically using the antibody LR1, caught during midmigration from the human olfactory placode to the basal forebrain. (Data from Schwanzel-Fukuda et al., 1996.)

Plate 12 (figure 8.6)   Immunocytochemically stained gonadotropin-releasing hormone (GnRH) neurons arrested in migration from the olfactory placode (which would appear below the bottom of this photograph) toward the human basal forebrain (which would appear above the top of this photograph). This is human tissue from an individual with genetic damage at Xp22.3, consistent with the development of Kallmann syndrome. In this Kallmann tissue, GnRH neurons never will reach the basal forebrain but instead are arrested as shown here, near the top of the olfactory apparatus, in a confused conglomeration. (From Schwanzel-Fukuda et al., 1989.)

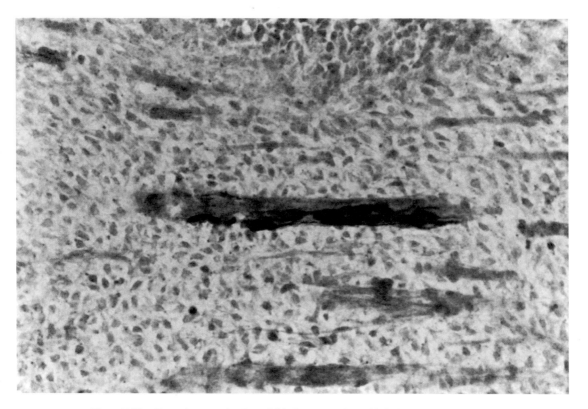

Figure 7.17 (For color reproduction of this figure see plate 10.) A GnRH neuron migrating up the nasal septum toward the brain during fetal development surrounded by Anosmin I immunoreactivity. (From Dellovade et al., in press.)

C. Sex Differences as Examples of Genetic Effects

The use of gene expression for nuclear hormone receptors illustrates certain principles of genetic effects on behavior (as spelled out). As a result, a more general treatment of genes and behavioral sex differences also can be considered.

1. In Lower Animals

Clearly, sex differences in animal brain and behavior, where mediated by hormonal differences, represent *indirect* effects of genes on behavior. The expression of the SRY gene, demonstrated by Lovell–Badge and his colleagues, during development leads to the subsequent expression of the gene for a Müllerian inhibiting substance, which in turn masculinizes primitive gonadal development (Haqq & Donahoe, 1998; Lee et al., 1996, 1997; Teixeira et al., 1996). Müllerian tract development is suppressed so that the cortex of the gonad cannot grow into an ovary. Instead, Wolffian tract development is favored in the primordial gonad, leading to growth of the medulla of the gonad, yielding testes. From this critical, genetically dependent step follow a panoply of hormonal changes.

Among these hormonal sex differences, most important for brain development is the fact that the normal genetic male will have testes that secrete testosterone. In the rat, exposure of the brain to testosterone during the neonatal period (from birth to 4 or 5 days postnatally) is sufficient for masculinizing many sexually differentiated behaviors and neuroendocrine functions (table 7.8). How does the neonatal hormone action work? Surprisingly, in the brain, testosterone is transformed chemically (aromatized) to produce estradiol, which in turn works through the ER. This is proved not only by ER blocker studies but by selective administration of ER antisense DNA to the neonatal hypothalamus (figure 7.18; McCarthy et al., 1993).

Therefore, the prevailing theory is that testicular androgens aromatized in brain work on the hypothalamus during brain development to masculinize endocrine controls and behavior. Notably, in songbirds, this theory may not be sufficient to explain song development (Arnold et al., 1996; Wade & Arnold,

Table 7.8 Neonatal androgens determine both sexual and nonsexual behaviors of adult rats

	Lordosis/mount ratio		Emotional/fear responses	
	With E	With E+P	% Emerging[a]	Open field[b]
Control females	43	67	65	4.3
Neonatally castrated males	35	53	36	3.6
Neonatally testosterone-injected females	5	9	21	2.0
Control males	4	5	17	2.7

E, estrogen; P, progesterone.
[a]In emergence test, less fearful rats emerge first.
[b]Mean internal squares entered, an index of fearlessness.
Source: From Pfaff and Zigmond, 1971.

1996) and, indeed, expression of the SRY gene itself in the brain could be involved, at least in birds. Nevertheless, the theory regarding the indirect developmental effects of androgens and their metabolites (supported earlier) accounts for a tremendous body of data in a wide variety of animals and humans (Goy & McEwen, 1980).

The obvious behavioral consequences of neonatal testosterone administration in rats are to abolish lordosis behavior and increase male-typical mounting behavior. In addition, a variety of sex-differentiated emotional behaviors are masculinized (see table 7.8; Pfaff & Zigmond, 1971). In summary, a wide range of endocrine consequences follow from expression of the SRY gene in animals and (see following section) in humans.

2. IN HUMANS

The range of human sexual roles is large and always has generated great popular interest. Indeed, the word *hermaphrodite* stems from the name *Hermes,* a masculine Greek god famous for his strength, and the name *Aphrodite,* known for her beauty. The hermaphrodite has anatomical features of both the male and the

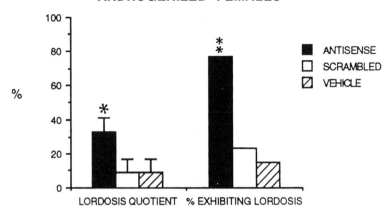

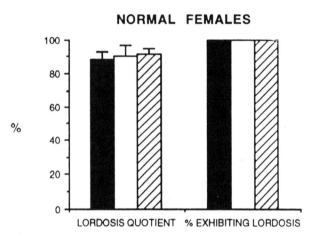

Figure 7.18   Neonatal female rats either had been given injections of testosterone 3 days after *birth* (androgenized females) or were given control injections (normal females). Within each of these two groups, some received hypothalamic microinjections of antisense DNA directed against the messenger RNA for the estrogen receptor (solid bars, antisense), a scrambled sequence control DNA (open bars, scrambled), or vehicle control (hatched bars, vehicle). Later, in adulthood, all females were tested for reproductive behavior under the influence of estrogen plus progesterone. Hypothalamic application of antisense DNA against ER messenger RNA actually reversed the testosterone effect in Androgenized Females and, as a control, did not affect behavior in the Normal Females. (From McCarthy et al., 1993.)

female, including both ovarian and testicular tissues. More concretely (Wilson et al., 1993, 1995), interruption of androgen actions throughout the body during human development disrupts normal masculinization of behavior.

In humans as in animals, testicular androgens are required not only for the differentiation of male sex organs but for behavioral changes during puberty and normal male sex drive. Here as elsewhere in this book, animal neuroendocrinology and neurobiology carries over to the explanation of human sexual behavior (see chapter 8).

Defects in this masculinization process follow obviously from abnormalities in the androgen receptor (AR). Inadequate AR causes ambiguity of the external genitalia and thus, abnormal sex rearing and absence of normal masculine role behavior. In this respect, the human syndrome represents our own species' version of the mouse testicular feminizing mutation syndrome (Attardi, 1978; Attardi et al., 1973; Ohno et al., 1973).

In addition, genetic abnormalities in the enzyme steriod 5-α-reductase (type 2), which converts testosterone to dihydrotestosterone (binding to AR), cause defects in normal masculinization. Because of peripheral genital changes, affected patients are raised as girls and assume typical female gender roles. Frequently, gender roles then are reversed again at puberty, depending on the culture in which the individual has been raised. Both these two conditions—the testicular feminizing mutation and the steroid reductase deficiency—illustrate the interactions of social considerations with the effects of hormonal and physical alterations during development.

In summary, genetic changes that disrupt the normal actions of androgens during development, through the AR, interfere with the development of normal male gender role behavior (see also figure 5.15).

D. SUMMARY

We have established that sex hormones can turn on specific genes at particular times in particular neurons which themselves are important for normal reproductive behavior. In turn, those gene products help to facilitate normal reproductive behavior. Moreover, in controlling sex behavior, nuclear hormone receptors, such as ER and TR, interact in a manner that reflects environmental changes and comprises a new level of neural integration.

Some gene effects on behavior are direct. Knocking out either the ER gene or the PR gene abolishes the facilitation by estrogen or progesterone, respectively, of female reproductive behavior. *How* does the ER gene act on behavior? By making a transcription factor which aids the synthesis of behaviorally important products. *How* does the TR-β gene act in this system? At least in part, by blocking ER function.

Other gene-behavior relations are indirect, the causal routes being quite complex. Many examples are found in the field of sexual differentiation of behavior, in animals and humans. The human condition, Kallmann's syndrome, offers a particularly complex illustration.

Comparisons of the results from our various experiments to date show that the effect of a particular gene on a specific behavior depends on the gender in which the gene is expressed, exactly when and where it is expressed, and the precise conditions of assay. In fact, the three-way *interaction* of genotype (G) with internal (*In*) with external (*Ex*) signals in directing behavior is demonstrated: In females (G) but not males, estrogens (*In*) allow somatosensory stimuli (*Ex*) to trigger lordosis behavior.

But what can be said about our human desires and feelings? Our minds?

8

Libido

The Problem of Sexual Excitation: "the accumulation of the sexual substances creates and maintains sexual tension . . . special chemical substances are produced . . . and then taken up in the blood stream and cause particular parts of the central nervous system to be charged with sexual tension . . . "

—S. Freud, *Three Essays on the Theory of Sexuality,* 1905

A. Freud and Libido

Already in his forties, Freud was in trouble. He had given up his early career as a neurologist, was an outsider in Viennese medical circles, and had not yet established himself solidly as a healer of minds. Nevertheless, during his forties and the next decade, the concepts he came up with, both from his treatment of patients and in correspondence with his circle of admirers, laid the groundwork for psychoanalysis for the next 50 years. Even then, his first public acclaim did not come from the European medical community but from the United States (Boorstin, 1983). Many of his findings and concepts are still much too complex for neurobiologists to confront. However, one central concept—

that of *libido*—is simple and primitive enough to be susceptible of genetic and molecular explanation.

Freud's concept of libido purposefully straddled the border between biological and psychological thought. In the simplest psychoanalytical terms, libido is defined as a force originating in physiological signals and acting on the mind. Freud's basic idea about the existence of a primitive sexual drive operating in the human psyche has received widespread acceptance from biologically inclined psychiatrists (Sulloway, 1979). Freud apparently saw no important differences between concepts of sexual drive in animals and the most primitive manifestations of libido as presented in psychoanalysis.

As concepts on the frontier between the somatic and the mental, "instinct" or "drive" comprised, for Freud, somatically determined demands made on the mind for psychic work. These demands constituted "pressures" or "forces" shaping mental events. Freud described pressure or force in terms of the notion of a quantifiable psychic energy. In this way, he attempted to provide for the translation of motivational forces from the body into motivational forces in the mind. These concepts bring together endogenously generated stimuli or excitation with their psychic concomitants, which consequently were invested with a mental energy or force. These psychic representatives could be inferred from the acts compelled by the drives (Freud, S., *Instincts and their Vicissitudes,* S.E. Volume 14 pp. 117-140). Early in this century, Freud failed in his attempts to explain psychological phenomena in terms of biological factors, but he maintained throughout his life that biological science eventually would provide the knowledge that would make another try useful and successful.

Modern psychoanalysts are properly cautious about any attempt to correlate biological with mental events. Nevertheless, all indications about the nature of estrogen and progesterone-dependent outputs from hypothalamic neurons point toward important hormonally influenced contributions to a *generalized drive state* that sets up behavioral dispositions in favor of reproduction (Pfaff & Peyser, in press). This accumulation of evidence now raises the possibility that neurobiological and molecular biological data are becoming available with enough precision and detail that we can begin to provide the biological foundations for certain aspects of Freud's concept of drive and its psychic energy.

The relation of Freud's ideas to modern neurophysiological projects is that he considered the sexual instinct as a composite of component instincts, explainable in physiological terms, that took their force from stimuli that originated in body organs or parts (Freud, 1905, *Three Essays on the Theory of Sexuality* S.E. Volume 7 pp. 125–245). Apparently, these simple energetic concepts of Freud's, such as drive or instinct, have the broad physiological character required for encompassing our new neuronal and molecular information.

The reasoning and data introduced in chapter 4 and elaborated in chapters 5 through 7 demonstrate clearly that estrogenic and progestin actions on hypothalamic neurons set up a general drive state. This notion, in turn, opens the possibility that we have discovered neurobiological and molecular biological foundations for the biological aspects of Freud's concept of instinct or drive (i.e., libido). Certainly, his original concepts have given us a place to start in linking the somatic to the mental, "building bridges to the psyche."

B. Can Studies of Libido Help to Approach One Component of the Mind-Body Problem?

Discussion of the mind-body problem, formerly dominated by philosophers and psychologists, have come to include neurophysiologists and other neurobiologists who are so impressed with the recent accumulation of data in the neurosciences that they want to try to approach the biological origins of consciousness. Respectable compilations of results have come under the rubric *Cognitive Neurosciences* (MIT Press, 1995). Still, the biological side of consciousness has remained an essentially philosophical topic (Chalmers, 1996; Dennett, 1996) occasioned by rather bitter debates (Penrose, 1989; Pinker, 1996).

Because of the controversies and disputes that have continued to characterize the purely philosophical approaches to this problem, it is obvious that only the simplest parts of the problem should be attacked using biological techniques: One should choose an aspect of mental life that is closest to being dominated by biological determinants. Strategically, in laying the groundwork for the neural and molecular explanation of Freud's concept of sexual drive, libido (already summarized) might be the best place to start. Precisely because libido has a hybrid character, being both a physiological and psychological concept, it represents the point of greatest potential equality between the physiological and psychological aspect. Therefore, one can argue that if the relevant neuroendocrine mechanisms really have been conserved adequately from animal brains into human brains (see following section), the demonstration of a biological explanation for a psychological concept actually might be achieved.

How far can a thorough reductionist approach to behavior take us, with detailed cellular and molecular techniques in play? And, how complex, subtle, and private might be the aspects of human behavior and mentation thus considered? Recognizing that the claim, the accumulation of data, and the ambition of this book are large indeed, we must, *pari passu,* state explicitly the limitations on this approach. Humans are not rats. We are not intending in this chapter or the foregoing to explain culturally rich aspects of romance or similar arenas of human social behavior. Rather, we are claiming to have delved into the most primitive, biologically based urges without which the more elevated steps of human sexual behaviors would not occur—lust rather than love. In doing so, we address the element of human motivation long validated by the drive theory of psychoanalysis, physiological psychology, and ethology.

C. BIOLOGICAL DOMAINS RELATED TO LIBIDO AND CONSERVED FROM ANIMAL BRAINS TO HUMAN BRAINS AND BEHAVIOR

Many features of neurobiological mechanisms, endocrine principles, and reproductive biology have remained the same among a variety of mammals and humans. As a result, one can argue easily that the conservation of these important brain mechanisms contributes to the explanation of libido.

General Conservation among Mammals

All mammals shared a common ancestor approximately 140 million years ago. A tremendous number of the physiological features have remained in place, as mammals evolved from the types of smaller quadrupeds (typically used in laboratories of experimental biology) to humans themselves. Overall, these simi-

----

larities are much more impressive than are the differences. After all, virtually all the major organs, sketal structure, and (most importantly) the means of reproduction have remained the same. Genomes are approximately the same size (as described in *Nature Biotechnology,* 14:1233–1239, 1996) and they contain large regions of chromsomes wherein genes are ordered in an identical fashion. Proteins that have similar functions between experimental laboratory rodents and humans usually have more than 90% identity in their amino acid sequences.

Moreover, the general tendency throughout nature is to conserve substances, physiological operations, and transformations once they have evolved to a biologically adaptive form. Logically, therefore, the most parsimonious approach is to assume that neuronal mechanisms of animal drive provide the primitive basis for the neural mechanisms of human drive. The effects of estrogens and androgens on sexual motivation—"lust"—in higher primates, including humans, have been published repeatedly (Fisher, in press). Therefore, given that we can explain hormonal, neuronal, and molecular bases of certain forms of animal reproductive behavior in considerable detail (chapter 4 through 7) we can infer that these fundamental investigations have a lot to do with the energetic concepts of human mind and behavior. From this point of view, the burden of proof is on those who claim that the biological basis of human drive is much different from what we have determined.

Beyond these more general arguments are many parallelisms between animals and humans in their reproductive endocrinology, biology, and behavior. In them, remarkable conservation of mechanisms can be illustrated as follows.

1. ENDOCRINE AND NEUROENDOCRINE

Steroid Hormones

Estrogens and progestins effective in evoking female-typical reproductive behavior, as well as androgens and their metabolites useful for stimulating male-typical behavior remain chemically identical between lower mammals and humans. In both cases (see later), androgens also may influence sex drive in females, and aromatization of androgens to estrogens remain important in the male. As the

———

steroids remain identical, one normally expects that neural mechanisms responding to them also would be very similar between animals and humans.

Hormone Receptor Chemistry

Likewise, the coding regions of the genes for steroid sex hormone receptors are conserved almost totally across mammalian species, leading to the inevitable conclusion that their chemical functions are essentially identical between animals and humans. Gene promoters for these same receptors are extremely similar between animals and humans, suggesting that, except for differences in detail, the regulation of gene expression for hormone receptors is very similar across a range of mammals, including humans.

Hormone Receptor Neuroanatomy

The basic limbic-hypothalamic system of estrogen receptor–containing cells and androgen receptor–containing neurons was discovered first in rats (Pfaff, 1968a; Pfaff & Keiner, 1973). This system has been conserved in considerable detail all the way from fish through primates (Morrell & Pfaff, 1978). Most exciting is the evidence (from the laboratory of Prof. Naomi Rance) that this same system appears in the human brain (figures 8.1 and 8.2). In some animals, extra groups of hormone-concentrating neurons also can be discerned, and these are related easily to details of sexual behavior in those species. The largest groups of neurons with the highest amounts of steroid receptors have been conserved remarkably well across mammals, even into the human brain.

2. HYPOTHALAMIC AND NEUROANATOMICAL

Hypothalamic Neuroanatomy

The fundamental neuroanatomy of the hypothalamus and its neuroendocrine and neuroanatomical connections, most closely related to libido, are conserved

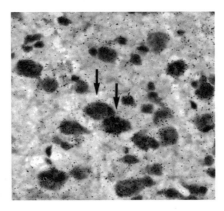

Figure 8.1   Small black grains over the cell bodies in the middle of this photomicrograph (arrows) demonstrate a positive in situ hybridization result: expression of estrogen receptor messenger RNA in the infundibular nucleus of human female hypothalamic tissue. (From Rance et al., 1990.)

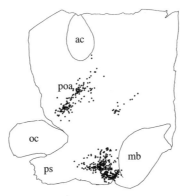

Figure 8.2   Microscopical map of neurons expressing estrogen receptor messenger RNA in a sagittal section of the human hypothalamus. Here, Rance has used a radioactively labeled cDNA probe directed against the messenger RNA for the human estrogen receptor and has used the technique of in situ hybridization to localize neurons expressing that messenger RNA in sections of both premenopausal and postmenopausal women who died suddenly from unexpected causes. The upper cluster of dots near the anterior commissure delineates a group of estrogen receptor–expressing neurons in the medial preoptic area. The lower cluster of dots identifies estrogen receptor neurons in the human infundibular nucleus, a region of the ventral hypothalamus that would correspond to the arcuate nucleus in lower mammals and in the adjacent ventromedial and ventral premammillary nuclei. Strikingly, the distribution published by Rance (1990) is perfectly homologous to the preoptic and ventral hypothalamic distributions in female rats (Pfaff & Keiner, 1973) and in rhesus monkeys (Pfaff et al., 1976). Thus, the ability of estrogen to turn on gene expression using the nuclear estrogen receptor in specific groups of preoptic and hypothalamic neurons is virtually identical across this range of animals and humans.

in the human brain to a remarkable degree. As we move from animal brain to human brain, cell groups remain recognizable: The arcuate nucleus, the ventromedial hypothalamic nucleus, the dorsomedial hypothalamic nucleus, the premammillary nuclei, the mammillary bodies, the very prominent paraventricular nucleus and supraoptic nuclei, and certain cell groups within the preoptic area remain essentially identical. Grouping of cells around the third ventricle are the same: The organum vasculosum of the lamina terminalis and the periventricular stratum are identical. Not only do neuroanatomical connections between the hypothalamus and the limbic system remain strong but the close anatomical relations with the midbrain central gray remain strong in the human brain. Of course, the important set of neuroendocrine connections to the median eminence (in humans named the *infundibulum*) remain in place, as do the details of the hypothalamic projections to and portal vessel communications to the posterior pituitary and anterior pituitary, respectively. The positioning of medial hypothalamic and preoptic groups between the long communicating systems of the medial forebrain bundle, the fornix, the mammillothalamic tract, the periventricular system and, dorsally, the major communicating systems to and from the thalamus likewise remain the same.

Neural Connections of Hormone-Responsive Neurons

Early on, cell groups of steroid sex hormone–concentrating neurons were noted to tend to project to other cell groups of hormone-concentrating neurons (Pfaff & Keiner, 1973). As neuroanatomical information became available in greater detail, this tendency was even more prominent (Cottingham & Pfaff, 1986). The heavily interconnected system of sex hormone–responsive cell groups within limbic and medial hypothalamic structures has remained substantially similar between animals and humans, even as other parts of the brain (e.g., the thalamus, cerebral cortex, and cerebellum) have changed greatly. Functional evidence of the importance of this similarity comes from the fact that across a wide variety of species, medial hypothalamic neurons are important for female-typical reproductive behavior, whereas medial preoptic neurons are important for male-typical behavior (Kelley & Pfaff, 1978). This conclusion is not limited to reproductive behavior but includes other aspects of drive. Hypothalamic damage is associated with changes in motivated behavior with respect to food intake as well (see, for example, Reeves & Plum, reviewed in Stellar, 1974). More generally, therefore, these primitive biologically based drives appear to have retained their animal mechanisms in the human hypothalamus.

Gonadotropin Release

The gonadotropin-releasing peptide is important because it governs all mammalian reproduction and, in fact, can facilitate mating behavior (Moss & McCann, 1973; Pfaff, 1973). Its behavioral facilitation is congruent with its control over reproduction elsewhere in the body. A surge of gonadotropin-releasing hormone [GnRH; luteinizing hormone releasing hormone (LHRH)] drives the ovulatory surge of luteinizing hormone in all species tested, from rats to humans (Moenter et al., 1991; Pau et al., 1993; Sarkar et al., 1976). The coding region of the GnRH gene is substantially the same between lower mammals and humans, and the decapeptide that is physiologically active is identical in animals and humans. Importantly, the histochemistry and neuroanatomical distribution of GnRH-expressing neurons are very similar between mammalian experimental animals and the human brain (figures 8.3 and 8.4 from the laboratories of Professors Naomi Rance and Joan King). Physiologically, the requirement for a pulsatile GnRH discharge into the portal circulation for ovulation in the genetic female is true in all the mammals studied. Thus, from all points of view, GnRH biology has been conserved from animal to human brain.

GnRH Neuron Migration

A startling discovery is that GnRH neurons are not born in the brain itself but instead are born in the olfactory epithelium and must migrate during development up the nose, along the bottom of the brain, and into the preoptic area

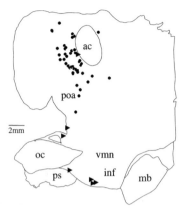

Figure 8.3   Microscopical mapping of neurons expressing the gene for gonadotropin-releasing hormone (GnRH) in a sagittal section of the human hypothalamus (Rance & Uswandi, 1996). Here, the mapping performed by Rance to chart the neurons using in situ hybridization for GnRH messenger RNA yields a distribution of GnRH gene expressing neurons in the same region of the brain as found in lower mammals. Across the range of all mammals studied, GnRH neurons can be found from the septum adjacent to the preoptic area, through the preoptic area itself, to the medial hypothalamus. The human distribution fits this perfectly. (See also Rance et al., 1994.)

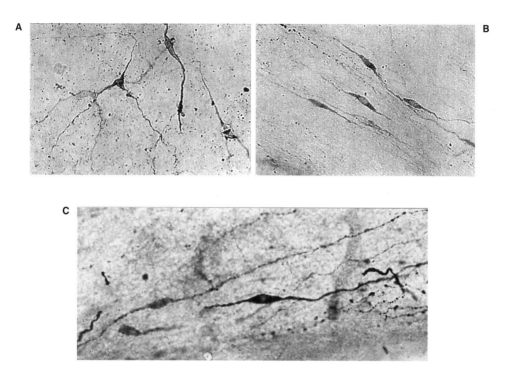

Figure 8.4   Gonadotropin-releasing hormone (GnRH) neurons in the human brain. (*A*) In the preoptic area of the human brain adjacent to the organum vasculosum of the lamina terminalis (OVLT), bipolar and tripolar GnRH neurons stained by immunocytochemistry. (*B*) Bipolar GnRH neurons in the medial basal human hypothalamus. (*C*) A well-stained luteinizing hormone–releasing hormone immunopositive cell body in the preoptic area. In general, in both their microscopical features and in their anatomical distribution, the population of human GnRH neurons is remarkably similar to that of GnRH neurons in lower animals. (Photomicrographs and data from the laboratory of Professor Joan King at Tufts University School of Medicine; Stopa et al., 1991; King et al., 1985.)

(Schwanzel-Fukuda & Pfaff, 1989). That discovery was made in the mouse. Subsequently, the GnRH neuronal migration has been confirmed in all vertebrate species studied, ranging from fish (Parhar et al., 1996) through human beings (figure 8.5) (Schwanzel-Fukuda et al., 1996). In fact, interruption of the migration in human beings accounts for Kallmann's syndrome, accompanied by a loss of libido (figure 8.6; Schwanzel-Fukuda et al., 1989).

3. MOLECULAR, NEUROBIOLOGICAL

Genes in the Brain

The fundamental structure of DNA and the organization of the promoters and coding sequences of genes expressed in the brain important for motivated behaviors remains in its elementary chemistry the same from animal brains to human brains.

Molecular Biology of Neurons

Everything known in the modern terms of molecular biology about the operation of transcriptional mechanisms and RNA processing indicates identity of mechanisms across mammalian species. Likewise, the chemical synthesis and functional operations of enzymes, structural proteins, and proteins produced for export again, in their modern understanding, appear in every respect identical among mammalian species.

Neurotransmitters and Neuropeptides

The fundamental chemistries of neurotransmitters and neuropeptides involved in basal forebrain function have by and large remained the same as we move from animal brain to human brain (e.g., the expression of enkephalins; figure 8.7). New neurotransmitters or neuropeptides were not just invented suddenly for human hypothalamic physiology. Moreover, in general terms, the neuroanatomy and histochemistry of these substances important for the control of reproduction have been conserved in all major respects.

Neurophysiology

The mechanisms of neural signaling by electrical action potentials and the resultant deposition of neurotransmitters and neuropeptides are so fundamentally similar among nerve cells of different species as to preclude any reason to believe that these elements of reproductive behavior mechanisms would be different between animals and humans. Likewise, synaptic mechanisms appear identical across a range of mammalian species.

Neuropharmacology

The pharmacology and endocrinology of reproductive behavior appears grossly similar between animals and humans. The role of testicular androgens is proved easily by castration studies in animals and by observing the absence of libido in eunuchs. In women, as in females from lower species, long-term absence of estrogens can reduce libido. Even the contributions of adrenal or ovarian androgens are parallel (figure 8.8; see later).

If the case for conservation can be made for normal sex drive, what can we say about hypersexual men? As has been rendered clear, some of these men and certain other sex offenders actually *want* castration or antiandrogen treatment as a strategy to reduce their libido and thereby to keep themselves out of trouble. Most to the point, as in lower animals, surgical castration, or treatment with such compounds as cyproterone acetate or synthetic progestins [e.g., Depo-Provera (medroxyprogesterone)], which block androgen action, can be effective. Furthermore, continuous treatment with a GnRH analog delivered on a time schedule to desensitize GnRH receptors in the human pituitary can reduce hypersexuality in male patients (Thibaut et al., 1994).

As a side point, the ability of mood-altering drugs to change sexual drive gives another line of evidence for the parallelism between the kinds of neural

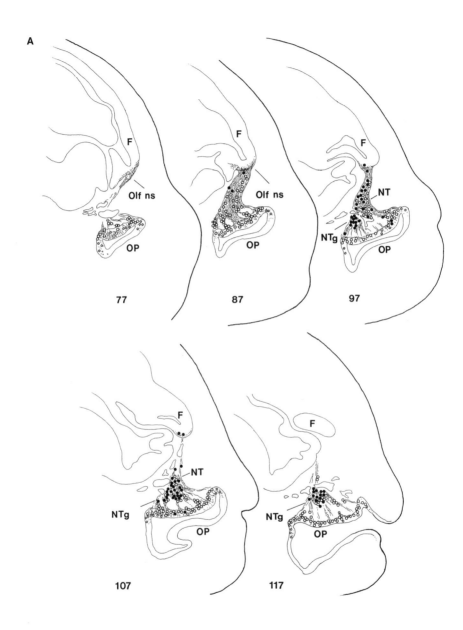

B

C

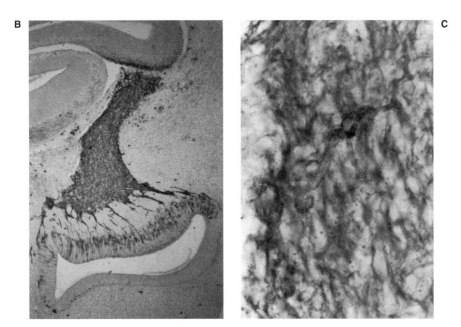

Figure 8.5   (For a color reproduction of this figure, see plate 11.) (*A*) Gonadotropin-releasing hormone (GnRH) neurons (small circles, both open and closed) during migration from the olfactory pit (OP) to the basal forebrain (F). Selected sagittal sections 77, 87, 97, 107, and 117, from human tissue 42 days post fertilization. Each circle represents a GnRH-expressing neuron. (Data from Schwanzel-Fukuda et al., 1996.) (*B*) Low-power photomicrograph corresponding to section 87. Even at low magnification, some of the red-brown-stained GnRH neurons are visible migrating from the olfactory pit (aperture at bottom) to the basal forebrain (*top*). (*C*) At higher magnification, red-brown-stained GnRH neurons, recognized immunocytochemically using the antibody LR1, caught during midmigration from the human olfactory placode to the basal forebrain. (Data from Schwanzel-Fukuda et al., 1996.)

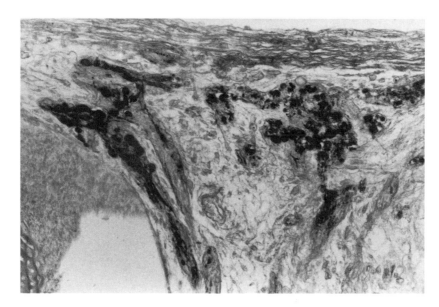

Figure 8.6 (For a color reproduction of this figure, see plate 12.) Immunocytochemically stained gonadotropin-releasing hormone (GnRH) neurons arrested in migration from the olfactory placode (which would appear below the bottom of this photograph) toward the human basal forebrain (which would appear above the top of this photograph). This is human tissue from an individual with genetic damage at Xp22.3, consistent with the development of Kallmann's syndrome. In this Kallmann tissue, GnRH neurons never will reach the basal forebrain but instead are arrested as shown here, near the top of the olfactory apparatus, in a confused conglomeration. (From Schwanzel-Fukuda et al., 1989.)

Figure 8.7 Computer-assisted mapping of the distribution of enkephalin-expressing cells in the human hypothalamus (from Sukhov et al., 1995). In coronal section (A) and in sagittal section (B), we see the results of in situ hybridization for gene expression for prepro-enkephalin in the human hypothalamus. Identification of enkephalin-expressing cells in the ventromedial nucleus, the dorsal medial nucleus, and tuberal cell groups nicely matches the mapping of enkephalin gene expression in the rat brain (Harlan & Pfaff, 1987). For this important opioid peptide, therefore, which bears on reproductive drive in the female (see chapter 7), the distribution of cells remains highly homologous between rat medial hypothalamus and human medial hypothalamus (from Sukhov et al., 1995, figures 7 and 8). For other neuropeptides as well, in the human infundibulum (e.g., substance P), that are important for female reproductive behavior, the distribution in the basal medial hypothalamus provides an excellent parallelism between animal brain and human brain (Rance & Young, 1991).

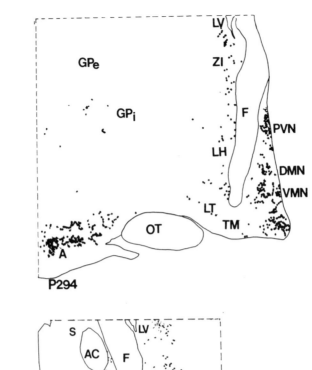

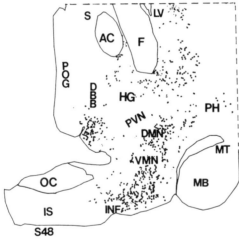

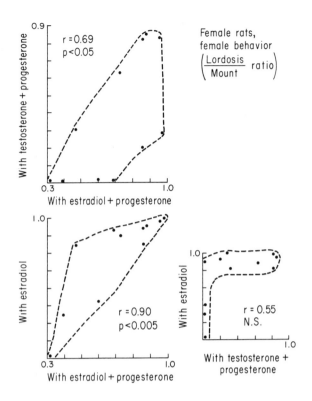

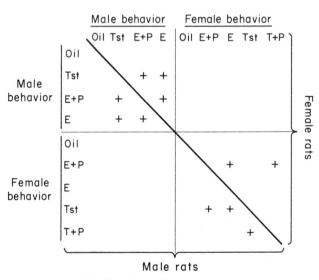

+ = Significant positive correlation
No significant negative ones occurred

mechanisms we study and human libido. Prozac (fluoxetine), a selective serotonin reuptake inhibitor, often reduces sex drive and readiness for orgasm in men and women, thus providing another mind-brain linkage in this domain of reproductive neuroendocrinology.

4. REPRODUCTIVE BIOLOGY

Biology of Sex Differences

The great ethologist E.O. Wilson (1978) has pointed out a host of sex differences retained from animal to human biology. Huge differences in size between female and male gametes, sex differences in the biological costs of bringing an infant to term and caring for it, differences in intraspecific aggression, and the like, have been retained in human biology.

Requirements for Fertilization

The fundamental requirements for reproduction, including uniting of sperm and egg, are as true for humans as for lower animals. The basic physiology and

Figure 8.8 (*A*) Female rats can respond to androgenic hormone, testosterone, with increased levels of lordosis behavior (Pfaff, 1970). In fact, there is a significant correlation between the individual female rats (each point = one female) that respond to testosterone and progesterone and those that respond to estradiol and progesterone (*upper left scattergram*). The correlation is not as good as the correlation between responses of individual females to estradiol and the responses to estradiol and progesterone (*lower left scattergram*). The ability of animals to respond with female-typical behavior to injected androgenic hormone provides another parallel with humans, in which androgens also have been connected with libido. (*B*) Among female rats, across several hormonal conditions, individual differences in tissue sensitivities to injected hormones affected the magnitude of lordosis behavior responses (Pfaff, 1970). Each plus sign indicates a pair of hormonal conditions in which the same rats that responded best to one hormone condition also responded best to the other, producing a positive and significant rank correlation. This was true not only for lordosis behavior ("female behavior") exhibited by female rats but also for malelike behavior exhibited by female rats (*upper left quadrant*).

anatomy required for successful copulation also remain the same from animals to humans. Pelvic thrusting by the male and axial muscle tension by the female, the requirement for penetration, and the consequent need for synchronization between female and male behavior all are shared by animal and human reproductive systems. In both cases, synchronizing reproductive behavior with the condition of the rest of the body and its environment are the same. In both lower mammals and humans, nutrition, water supply, salt balance, and a "nesting" domicile all must be adequate, an attractive mating partner must be available, and a permissive environmental temperature and a relative absence of stress are requisites. In both animals and humans, the basic muscular and autonomic reflexes underlying erection in the male are fundamentally the same (Meisel & Sachs, 1994). So when we say about a crude, sexually active guy, "He's a real animal," we just might mean it!

5. ANDROGENS IN FEMALES

Even unusual or unexpected features of sex drive in females can carry over from animal behavior to human behavior. Strikingly, androgen treatment of ovariectomized female rats, followed by progesterone supplementation, could induce lordosis behavior in a reliable manner (Pfaff, 1970). In addition, in female rhesus monkeys, androgens (perhaps from the adrenal glands) were shown by Doris Zumpe and Richard Michael to render the female interested in or receptive toward the male. Equally striking, therefore, is not only that androgens are important for male libido in humans (Alexander et al., 1997) but also that androgens potentially of both adrenal and ovarian origins heighten women's sexual interest. Coexpression of androgen receptor and estrogen receptor in the same nerve cells might be involved here (Wood & Newman, 1995). In any case, along this unusual dimension of androgenic effects on female libido, extrapolation from animal behavior data to human behavior again has been justified.

6. SEX DIFFERENCES IN AGGRESSION

Even a casual acquaintance with the literature on mouse behavior demonstrates clearly that males are more aggressive than are females (Moyer, 1976; van Oort-

186

merssen & Bakker, 1991). The same is true with other experimental animals. Violence in human beings, extreme aggression even to the point of criminality, displays the same sex differences. Murder of unrelated males not only is perpetrated almost exclusively by males but the curve plotting the frequency of murders as a function of age is constant across cultures and is correlated closely with testosterone levels. Therefore, this type of male-initiated violence can be seen as having a biological basis probably dependent on androgens. Violence within the family virtually always is initiated by males (see Understanding and Preventing Violence, National Academy of Sciences Press, 1994). Crimes of sexual violence are so predominantly male that some municipalities provide no facilities for housing females who commit such crimes. Again, therefore, animal behavior data and likely mechanisms carry over to human behavior.

7. IMPLICATION

Faced with the large number of neurobiological and endocrine mechanistic similarities between a variety of mammals and humans, and the two additional domains of data just quoted, we have two choices. Either we can assume that nature, having evolved a set of mechanisms for mammalian reproductive behavior that worked very well, *threw away* all those mechanisms and independently evolved a new set of mechanisms that produce similar behavioral features *or,* as in a wide variety of other situations, mechanisms were *conserved* as we moved from mammalian neuroendocrine systems into the neural and endocrine mechanisms that govern the biological side of human libido. Those who study primate reproductive behavior long have held the latter opinion on this point (Maslow, 1936). They not only could see the similarities between lower primate behavior and normal human behavior but could see parallelisms between animals and humans in the so-called perversions (Maslow, 1936), and strongly urged, therefore, an understanding of the varieties of human sexual escapades in light of biological mechanisms that exist as well in lower primates. More generally, that highly evolved mechanisms of the sort discussed here would simply be discarded in nature seems wasteful and unlikely. Therefore, as we strive toward neurobiological summaries that unite certain features of animal and human behavior, we conclude that important features of the mechanisms described for female animal sex drive (chapters 4 through 7) apply importantly to the biological side of human female libido as well. Correspondingly, as the mechanisms for male-typical sex behavior become clearer (e.g., Meisel & Sachs, 1994), the same argument should apply to men.

D. SUMMARY

A large number of neurobiological, endocrine, physiological, and molecular mechanisms related to libido have remained the same between a variety of mammals and humans, valid "from mouse to Madonna." The logical inference is that in all important respects, the neural and endocrine mechanisms underlying sex drive that we have discovered in the animals used for physiological experiments apply also to human beings. This conclusion would apply to the elementary biological side of a fundamental human emotion—sexual desire—but not to the important cultural, nonhormonal influences.

Thus, in women, the physiological underpinnings of libido in its biological aspects should depend on estrogenic actions on preoptic area and hypothalamic neurons. As a result, gene expression (see chapters 5 and 7) for progesterone receptor, such opioid peptides as enkephalins, and such neuropeptides as oxytocin *and* its receptor will be elevated. Heightened electrical activity in medial hypothalamic neurons will affect the performance of a phylogenetically ancient spine-brainstem-spine circuit (see chapter 6) that controls axial musculature and coordinated autonomic reflexes.

Again, the caution is that we are providing an explanation only of the most primitive component of human sex drive which then is sculpted by the overwhelming cultural forces that shape or suppress libido.

All the neurobiological, molecular, endocrine, and behavioral data from chapters 4 through 8 combine to form a tightly reasoned argument that can be recapitulated, along with its implications, in the next chapter.

9

FROM MOLECULAR AND NEURAL FACT
TO BEHAVIORAL EXPLANATION

That Love is all there is,
Is all we know of Love;
It is enough, the freight should be
Proportioned to the groove.

—Emily Dickinson, "1765"

A. DRIVE, MOTIVATION

A major problem in neurobiology is to figure out why humans or animals do anything at all. What *motivates* behavior? The simplest and most practical way to discover neurobiological mechanisms is to explain the "lowest drives," which have an obvious biological component. With the findings described in chapters 4 through 8 and summarized here, we provide an explanation of what turns an inactive female animal with no sex drive into an animal that will show both active courtship and mating behaviors. The explanation (1) starts with the consequences of hormone receptor occupation in the brain, (2) moves on to elevated expression of specific genes in specific neurons, and (3) shows how altered hypothalamic readouts are manifested in behavioral changes (see chapter 6) via a thoroughly documented neuronal circuit.

The concept of drive is absolutely necessary in a rigorous logical sense to explain altered behavioral responses to constant stimuli in a constant environment. The basic neurobiological explanations for these primitive drives are likely to apply also to humans.

The two-component theory of drive would state that drives can both energize and direct behavior. At the neural and molecular level, the simplest behavioral phenomenon to tackle is the energization of behavior by a specific biochemical trigger. We know that steroid hormones can impressively turn on mating behaviors. Through their actions on ascending arousal mechanisms and preoptic locomotor-related neurons, estrogens drive courtship behaviors. Additionally, through their actions on the enkephalin gene in ventromedial hypothalamic neurons, estrogens can produce a partial analgesia that, through descending pathways (e.g., periaqueductal gray), permits lordosis behavior (Bodnar et al., in press). Energization of reproductive behaviors depends on the order of hormone administration, its duration, and the pattern of hormone metabolism. All these principles apply to human behavior but, for humans, hormones account for a smaller percentage of the determination of behavior.

With respect to brain mechanisms of motivation, the female rat and mouse sexual behavior systems have proved fairly amenable to investigation—neural circuit determined and molecular mechanisms pinpointed—because of their relative simplicity and because of their hormonal dependence. Now, they serve as a well-defined platform of knowledge from which to launch deeper behavioral analyses (e.g., on the most general features of arousal) and molecular analyses (e.g., on the promoters of hormone-dependent genes in neurons).

B. Mechanisms

1. Receptors

How do hormones influence motivation and behavior? Steroid hormones circulate in the blood and flood the brain but are retained in neurons only in the presence of hormone-specific receptors, nuclear proteins that mediate hormone-dependent transcription. During the golden age of molecular endocrinology, while Elwood Jensen, Bert O'Malley, and their colleagues were elucidating the receptor proteins and Pierre Chambon, Ron Evans, and their colleagues elucidating hormone receptor genes, we have been working out the central nervous system and limbic-hypothalamic systems that respond to sex hormones in a behaviorally important fashion. Using both hormone-binding techniques and in situ hybridization for hormone receptor gene products, we discovered the target neurons for estrogens and androgens in a system of ancient limbic system structures and medial hypothalamic cell groups. We were fascinated that the small groups of hypothalamic and limbic neurons thus pinpointed are themselves heavily interconnected. Further, these hormone-binding nerve cell groups direct hormone-dependent sex behavior.

The limbic-hypothalamic system of sex hormone–binding neurons discovered in rats has been replicated and extended for every vertebrate studied, from fish to human beings.

2. NEURAL CIRCUIT

What is the circuit through which hormone-activated neurons control hormone-dependent behavior? Summarized in chapter 6, it begins with cutaneous receptors and lumbar spinal responses to behaviorally sufficient stimuli from the male. The ascending side of the obligatory supraspinal loop runs in the anterolateral columns and terminates in the medullary reticular formation, lateral vestibulospinal nucleus, and midbrain central gray. Hormone-activated hypothalamic efferents have their impact on the midbrain central gray and surrounding midbrain neurons. Central gray efferents facilitate medullary reticulospinal systems that synergize with the lateral vestibulospinal system to turn on the axial motoneurons the output of which activates lordosis behavior.

This neural circuit was the first described for a vertebrate behavior and proves the possibility of discovering a neural circuit for a mammalian behavioral response (figure 9.1). The neural circuit for lordosis behavior divides nicely into

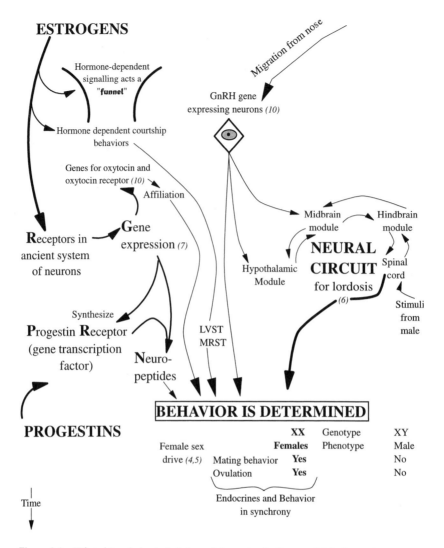

Figure 9.1 What drives behavior? A few of the major findings established in individual research articles and reviewed in this book are summarized here in schematic form. Gene expression clearly affects reproductive behavior during development (XX vs XY) and in adulthood. Early events tend to appear toward the top of the page, later events toward the bottom. Events flow from upper left to bottom right. Chapters are represented by small numbers in italics. Figure 9.2 presents a broader biological picture that includes these mechanisms. (GnRH, gonadotropin-releasing hormone; LVST, lateral vestibulospinal tract; MRST, medullary reticulospinal tract.)

modules, each with its own job and each matching a recognizable embryological subdivision of the neuraxis.

The principle established here is that a discoverable neural circuit underlies an integral mammalian behavior. In this circuit, natural biochemicals (hormones) working in specific parts of the brain cause changes in behavioral disposition. Reproductive behavior is determined by estrogen and progestin effects emanating from medial hypothalamic neurons interacting with specific ascending somatosensory signals.

Thus, this mechanism provides for the biologically sensible interaction of environmental stimulus with hormone effect. Two special features of this mechanism show a type of "orchestration" in this system in which earlier responses set up the system for later responses. First, over a long period before actual mating behavior, hormone-dependent communications between male and female comprise a "hormone-dependent behavioral funnel" that brings reproductively competent conspecifics together. Second, in the female, the consequences of courtship behaviors for the lateral vestibulospinal system raise excitability in the lordosis behavior circuit.

C. Genes

1. Hormone Influence on Gene Expression in Brain

Estrogens can turn on at least six neurochemical systems in hypothalamic neurons the products of which are important for lordosis behavior. These products include the gene for the progesterone receptor (PR), the gene for the opioid peptides *met*-enkephalin and *leu*-enkephalin (and for their delta opioid receptor), alpha-adrenergic receptors, muscarinic cholinergic receptors, the oxytocin gene and the gene for its receptor, and gonadotropin-releasing hormone (GnRH) and the gene for its receptor. At a number of different levels of molecular, neural, and behavioral analyses (see figures 7.1 and 7.3), the estrogen effects on the PR gene and preproenkephalin gene form a well-integrated set of mechanisms leading from hormone effect toward behavior (see figures 7.1 and 7.3). For oxytocin, enkephalins, and GnRH, the opportunity for *multiplicative* effects of hormones on a given neurochemical system (ligand effect × receptor effect) is obvious.

The principle is that estrogen turns on the gene for PR, a nuclear protein acting as a transcriptional activator. The PR gene product is important subsequently for lordosis behavior. This finding provides the first example of stimulation of a specific transcription factor in brain required for the facilitation of a specific behavior.

2. GENES DIRECTING BEHAVIOR

Some very clear gene effects on lordosis behavior are *direct*. Work with estrogen receptor (ER) knockout mice and PR knockout mice proves the roles of these genes in reproductive behavior in adult females.

Other equally clear gene effects on reproductive behaviors are *indirect* (chapter 7). The most blatant example comes from sex differences, in which the SRY gene product eventually leads to a host of behavioral alterations under the general rubric *masculinization* or *defeminization* of brain and behavior. A trickier example relates to our GnRH neuronal migration from the olfactory placode and explains the loss of libido in men with Kallmann's syndrome. Indeed, hypogonadal animals and people *can* manage the motor responses involved in sexual behavior because, in the manner of a "control experiment," they can respond to exogenous steroid sex hormone treatment. Thus, the reason for their loss of libido truly is that GnRH neurons are not in position to govern the pituitary that in turn governs the gonads.

From this work, at least three lessons about genetic effects of behavior have emerged. First, the effect of a given gene on a particular behavior can depend on the gender in which that gene is expressed (see chapter 7). Second, the effect can depend on exactly when and exactly where in the brain it is expressed. Finally, because of complex interactions with environment, the effect can depend exquisitely on the conditions of assay.

In sum, what now can be seen is how specific gene products operate in specific parts of the central nervous system to govern specific behaviors in experimental animals and in humans. In turn, the neural circuit explains how gene products are "read out" into behavioral results (see Mechanisms and chapter 6).

D. SYMPHONY

Especially for the female, whose biological costs for engaging in reproduction are remarkable, courtship and copulatory behaviors must be in harmony with aspects of her environment that are either permissive or forbidding. These include food supply, water, salt, environmental temperature, stress, length of day, time of day, nesting material, and the like, all in addition to communication signals coming from an adequate mating partner. How are the neural mechanisms for behavior orchestrated with these environmental factors?

We have seen how the biological requirements for adaptive sex behavior are met by at least three types of mechanisms: Neuropeptides by their very nature are essentially integrative (see also chapter 10). They can achieve a virtual symphony between the brain and the rest of the body. Second, neural interactions between internal (hormonal) and external signals guarantee behavioral reactions appropriate to the environment. Finally, we have shown integration through the competition and cooperation of transcription factors in the nuclei of hypothalamic neurons (figure 9.2).

1. HYPOTHALAMIC NEUROPEPTIDES

Some features of the orchestration of behavior with environmental limits simply depend on controls over the synthesis and release of neuropeptides, which then essentially embody an integrative role. For example, once the GnRH-producing neurons have reached their final neuroanatomical positions in the basal forebrain, the GnRH promoter responds to environmental signals such as stress. Controlled by such signals, the release of GnRH then serves to synchronize pituitary function and gonads (through release into the portal vasculature) with reproductive behavior (through release in the hypothalamus and midbrain)

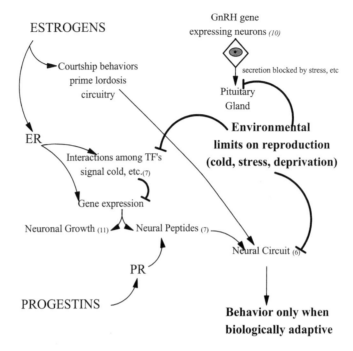

Figure 9.2   A virtual symphony of neural and endocrine mechanisms not only orchestrates the performance of reproductive behavior but also ensures that obvious biological requirements for the adaptiveness of reproduction (biological "axioms") are met. Many of the findings established by articles in the primary literature are reviewed in chapters 6 and 7. Chapters are denoted by small numbers in italics. The detailed mechanisms of figure 9.1 fit within this picture. (→, positively affects; ⊣, inhibits; ER, estrogen receptor; PR, progestin receptor; GnRH, gonadotropin-releasing hormone; TF, transcription factor.)

(Pfaff, 1973; see also chapter 10). Overall, therefore, steroid sex hormones and neuropeptides such as GnRH achieve a symphonic arrangement of environment, behavior, and the peripheral endocrine preparations for reproduction.

2. INTERNAL × EXTERNAL SIGNALS

The neural circuit revealed for lordosis behavior provides multiple opportunities for the interactions of peripheral sensory signals from the environment (prominent at the spinal cord level) with the descending effects of estrogens and progestins operating in hypothalamic neurons. Not just with behavioral assays but with molecular assays, the ability of painful stimuli, for example, to influence relevant neuronal responses to a sex hormone is clear. Of course, the most massive interaction is the obvious one between cutaneous signals from the male mating partner (an environmental reality) and the internal signals from the ovaries, estradiol and progesterone. At this level, the problem of how to understand [internal × environmental] integration has been solved.

3. INTERACTIONS AMONG TRANSCRIPTION FACTORS

For small rodents, which have a high surface-to-volume ratio, environmental cold is a terribly important signal helping to govern reproduction. Cold temperatures raise circulating thyroid hormone levels. In turn, liganded thyroid hormone receptors (TRs) can displace ERs bound to their cognate DNA estrogen response elements in the nuclei of hypothalamic neurons. As a consequence, estrogen-dependent transcription, as can be important for reproductive behavior, is disrupted. In fact, estrogen-facilitated lordosis behavior is reduced by exogenous and endogenous thyroid hormones. This series of mechanisms unites a biologically important environmental factor with a molecular mechanism in a well-studied neuroendocrine circuit. It shows how a DNA-binding and transcriptional interference can mediate an environmental limitation on a molar mammalian behavior.

Even beyond lordosis behavior mechanisms, thyroid hormones can influence responses to estrogens in the rat pituitary and reproductive seasonality in birds and sheep and can affect the menstrual cycle in female patients.

The foregoing processes highlight the principle that *cooperation and competition among transcription factors now is shown to comprise a new level of neuronal integration.* Putting questions of physiological integration into historical perspective illustrates that the first decade of the twentieth century was good for endocrinologists and neurophysiologists. After all, Bayliss and Starling in that decade did the experiments and thinking leading to modern endocrinology, and Sir Charles Sherrington, in his 1906 book *The Integrative Action of the Nervous System,* set the problem for the neurobiologists of this century.

At a *first level of investigation,* neurobiologists during all of the twentieth century have been solving Sherrington's problem by appealing to the complexities of neuroanatomy, synaptic connections, and electrophysiology to explain mechanisms of behavior. Then, at a *second level of investigation,* during the last 30 years, the increasingly sophisticated tools of neurochemistry and histochemistry have presented many facts about the dynamics of neurotransmitters and neuropeptides that reveal a corresponding type of neuronal integration. This progression has allowed opportunities for a new type of explanation of behavior to be superimposed upon the first.

Now, a *new, third level of investigation* exemplified in this book through the use of molecular biological techniques shows that the interactions among transcription factors in the nuclei of hypothalamic neurons—be they cooperative, as with ER and PR, or competitive, as with ER and TR—actually embody a novel form of neuronal integration. This type of molecular approach supplies explanations for behavior that are to be superimposed on the first two.

More generally, the coordination of internal and external signals, the biology of certain neuropeptides, and the exciting new interactions among transcription factors show us how order emerges in the world of the nervous system and behavior. A sufficiently simple behavioral response, driven by simple steroid hormones whose receptors are transcription factors, all have allowed us to see how behavior can be orchestrated to fit its environment.

E. Libido

What parts of these neural and endocrine explanations apply to human behavior? Chapter 8 presented a very large number of molecular, endocrine, neural, and behavioral dimensions in which Mother and Father Nature had conserved their successfully evolved approaches to the adaptive control of reproduction and had kept them the same from animal brain to human brain. These dimensions included (but were not limited to) the preservation in human biology of the steroid hormones themselves, the molecular biology and chemistry of their receptors, the neuroanatomy and connections of neurons with hormone receptors, the anatomy of certain neuropeptide-expressing neurons, basic features of medial hypothalamic anatomy and physiology, elementary mechanisms of transcriptional control and the coding sequences on DNA itself, fundamental electrophysiology and synaptic physiology, and (more broadly) the limitations on reproductive biology and the anatomy and physiology of copulatory behaviors.

The inference here is that mechanisms of neural integration and hormonal control evident in reductionistic studies of lower animal sexual behavior must apply to the explanations of the biological side of human libido, the primitive physiological component of human sexual motivation. Because of the marked parallelisms in some features of primitive reproductive behaviors and striking conservation of the neural and endocrine mechanisms controlling them, we propose an extension of the tremendous body of work on animal neuroendocrine and sex behavior mechanisms to the biological understanding of human libido.

Obviously, the tremendously greater sensory capacities and response repertoires of humans and the even greater opportunities for connectivity and integration imply that nonhormonal and non-mate-driven stimuli will play a greater role in humans. Our culture influences reproduction to an extent never seen in experimental animals. So, do we reduce ourselves to "Chemical Man and Chemical Woman"? Only to the extent that primitive endocrine signals working through ancient limbic and hypothalamic circuitry—thus to control the biological side of our libido—can at the same time grab control of our minds. All we can claim is to have discovered how molecular, endocrine, and neurobiological mechanisms contribute to the biological side of a thorough explanation of basic human instincts.

III

BEYOND SEX: GLOBAL ACTIONS OF HORMONES ON BRAIN

Sex hormone effects on the brain are not limited to simple sex behaviors and sex drives. The same hormones, using some of the same cellular mechanisms, can affect broad classes of behaviors. In at least one case, the same neuropeptide—oxytocin—both can participate in specific lordosis behavior mechanisms and can influence a more general behavioral tendency toward affiliation. Finally, estrogens also can stimulate neuronal growth in a manner that may be important for the sex drives treated heretofore but also for cognition.

10

Affiliation versus Aggression: Oxytocin versus Vasopressin

What do I care how much it may storm?
I've got my love to keep me warm . . .

—Irving Berlin, from "On the Avenue," 1936

Throughout this book, the major theme has been to explain a specific form of sex drive, to implicate interesting cellular and molecular mechanisms, and to show the wide applicability of these mechanisms across a range of mammalian animals. Indeed, the neuropeptide oxytocin is involved centrally in lordosis behavior circuitry, but its roles are not limited to one particular behavioral response. Here, we consider its more general importance in a variety of social behaviors. Especially interesting is the contrast with a chemically similar neuropeptide, vasopressin (AVP).

A. Physiology

Oxytocin and AVP are neuropeptides that evolved from the ancient precursor vasotocin, common in fish (figure 10.1). Chemically, they retain great similarity, seven of their nine amino acids remaining the same and both neuropeptides

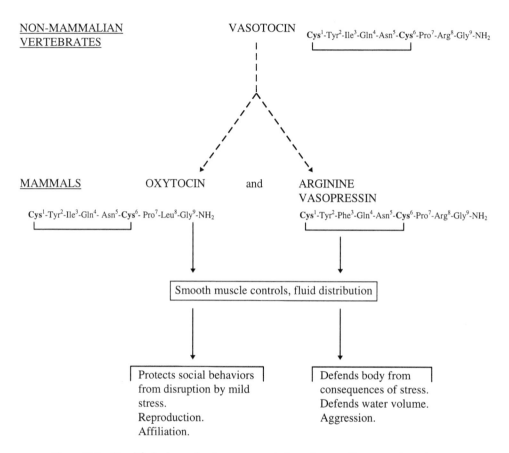

NON-MAMMALIAN VERTEBRATES

VASOTOCIN Cys^1-Tyr^2-Ile^3-Gln^4-Asn^5-Cys^6-Pro^7-Arg^8-Gly^9-NH_2

MAMMALS   OXYTOCIN   and   ARGININE VASOPRESSIN

Cys^1-Tyr^2-Ile^3-Gln^4- Asn^5-Cys^6- Pro^7-Leu^8-Gly^9-NH_2 Cys^1-Tyr^2-Phe^3-Gln^4-Asn^5-Cys^6-Pro^7-Arg^8-Gly^9-NH_2

Smooth muscle controls, fluid distribution

Protects social behaviors from disruption by mild stress.
Reproduction.
Affiliation.

Defends body from consequences of stress.
Defends water volume.
Aggression.

Figure 10.1 Simplified scheme for the recent evolution of mammalian oxytocin and vasopressin. A much broader range of early vertebrate and prevertebrate 9–amino acid peptides has also been explored from a molecular and evolutionary point of view (Acher, 1993; Heierhorst et al., 1989, 1993; Morley et al., 1990). Though some physiological functions of oxytocin and vasopressin have remained similar, in view of their chemical similarities, the differences in the effects of these neuropeptides on social behaviors have been quite surprising.

retaining the same disulfide bond. Indeed, some of their functions also remain similar, related to the stimulation of smooth muscles, water balance, and such major biological events as giving birth and responses to stress. If we follow Hans Selye (1974) in defining stress as a nonspecific response of the body to any demand made on it, we can begin to distinguish the functions of AVP from those of oxytocin (Carter & Altemus, 1997). AVP defends the body against severe stress by supporting aggressive responses and by enforcing restoration of water balance. Oxytocin protects normal social responses, especially in the female (Carter et al., 1997), from interruption by low-level, mild social stress.

For two peptides chemically so similar, the functional differences are surprising. AVP not only facilitates offensive aggression toward an intruder (Ferris & Delville, 1994) in a manner that depends on testosterone (Delville et al., 1996) but it greatly stimulates aggressive social signals, such as flank marks (Ferris, 1992). Within the hypothalamus, AVP is released in response to emotional stress (Wotjak et al., 1996). Aggressive responses to stress may have derived from the ancient functions of arginine vasotocin, which determined masculine aggressiveness in fish.

In dramatic contrast, oxytocin is the neurohormone of affiliation and love: maternal behavior and positive social responses (Insel & Shapiro, 1992a,b). The evidence from several zoological forms and many laboratories on this point has been so overwhelming that entire books have been devoted to its exposition (Carter et al., 1997; Pedersen et al., 1992). Estrogen-primed female voles receiving oxytocin in the cerebral ventricles showed more friendly social contacts and reduced aggressive responses when tested with a male partner (Carter et al., 1992). Emotionally neutral or positive social contacts and investigative responses in both genders (but especially in the female) depend on oxytocin (Witt, 1997). In fact, oxytocin exerts an anxiolytic action that depends on contemporaneous estrogen treatment (McCarthy et al., 1996, 1997). In doing so, oxytocin protects such instinctive behaviors as maternal and sexual responses from disruption by mild stress (McCarthy et al., 1991).

The protection by oxytocin of adaptive reproductive behaviors may be especially important, as some biologists feel that sexual behaviors set the paradigm for a broad variety of social behaviors. The dependence of certain maternal and reproductive responses on oxytocin carries through to human beings as well. Likewise, AVP functions are just as important for human health as they are for water balance in experimental animals (Gross et al., 1993).

Molecular evidence for the necessity of oxytocin receptor gene expression in the support of female reproductive behavior is especially clear. Antisense DNA against oxytocin receptor messenger RNA (mRNA) significantly reduced lordosis behavior (figure 10.2) if it was delivered to the ventromedial hypothalamus (McCarthy et al., 1994). The reversibility of the effect and the inclusion of control behavioral responses showed that the antisense DNA effect was not due to simple damage of hypothalamic neurons. In agreement with the antisense DNA results, an oxytocin receptor antagonist decreases estrogen-stimulated lordosis behavior (Witt & Insel, 1991, 1992).

1. PRINCIPLES OF NEUROPEPTIDE ACTION

Obviously, *the effect of a neuropeptide depends on how much already has been released.* In a normal physiological context, this principle refers to the major phenomenon of desensitization. After initial peptide action, receptors and their coupling are downregulated. In an experimental pharmacological context, this principle means that getting sensible results depends on application to receptors where the neuropeptide normally belongs but currently is in short supply.

More subtly, *the effect of a neuropeptide depends on the conditions of assay,* not only the genetic background of the test animal but also the degree of environmental stress. For example, Susan Fahrbach et al. (1986) discovered that the effect of oxytocin to facilitate maternal behavior depended on the degree of stress placed on the maternal female. If the female were totally comfortable "at home," she did not need experimentally applied oxytocin to be maternal. If instead she was highly stressed by a very novel environment, oxytocin would not help. Finally, if she had a chance to reduce stress by becoming familiar with the novel environment, the robust action of oxytocin to improve her maternal performance was revealed. Thus, even as oxythocin protects the instinctive

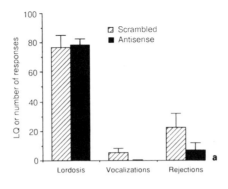

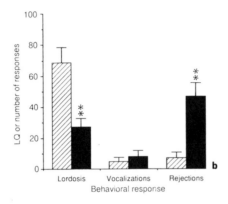

Figure 10.2   The reduction of female sexual behavior (lordosis quotient) caused by antisense DNA against oxytocin receptor messenger RNA (microinjected into ventromedial hypothalamus) was specific to the hormonal pretreatment used. (*a*) Female rats were pretreated with both estradiol and progesterone. Under this condition, the antisense DNA–treated females obtained the same results as did the "scrambled-sequence" controls. (*b*) Two weeks later, the same females were pretreated with estradiol only. Now, the antisense DNA against oxytocin receptor (microinjected into the ventromedial hypothalamus) significantly reduced lordosis behavior and significantly increased rejection behaviors as compared to the "scrambled-sequence" controls (From McCarthy et al., 1994.)

behavior from mild stress, that same mild stress permits the discovery of the oxytocin effect.

B. MOLECULAR BIOLOGY

Both oxytocin and AVP were cloned by Professor Dietmar Richter at the University of Hamburg. Gene expression for oxytocin and for the oxytocin receptor are both elevated in specific subsets of neurons by estradiol (for references see Bale & Dorsa, 1997; Dellovade et al., 1998; Quiñones-Jenab et al., in press). Because both the ligand and its receptor are increased, the two estrogen effects should *multiply* each other for a powerful behavioral effect.

Even though large-scale dissections of hypothalamic tissue failed to show a large hormone effect on oxytocin mRNA, a more painstaking cell-by-cell approach using in situ hybridization revealed a significant estrogen effect in a subset of hypothalamic paraventricular nucleus neurons (figure 10.3) (Chung et al., submitted). In particular, estrogen increased oxytocin mRNA in the portion of the paraventricular nucleus with cells projecting to the lower brainstem and spinal cord (i.e., the cell group most likely to be relevant for the control of behavior). Moreover, work with thyroidectomized rats demonstrated an additional condition on the estrogen effect. High thyroid hormone levels militated against an estrogen effect, whereas it was robust in thyroidectomized females (figure 10.4; see also figure 7.11; Dellovade et al., in press).

A long series of neurochemical experiments showed that estrogen could increase oxytocin binding in the ventromedial hypothalamus, precisely where it could act to facilitate oxytocinergic promotion of lordosis behavior. The pioneering work of Jack Elands with Professor Ron DeKloet was extended by H. Corini and M. Schumacher as well as by Al Johnson in the McEwen laboratory at Rockefeller University. Especially since the promoter of the rat oxytocin receptor gene revealed a functional estrogen response element (Bale & Dorsa, 1997), a reasonable adjunct was to look for a hormone effect on oxytocin receptor gene expression in hypothalamic neurons. Vanya Quiñones-Jenab et al. (1997) used in situ hybridization to do so and found a significant estrogen stimulation of this gene in the ventromedial hypothalamus (VMH)

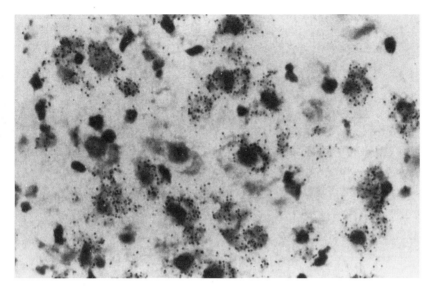

Figure 10.3   In situ hybridization for the messenger RNA (mRNA) for oxytocin in neurons of the paraventricular nucleus (PVN) of the hypothalamus. Sookja Kim Chung, working with McCabe and Haldar, used this technique to identify oxytocin gene–expressing neurons (grains over cell bodies), to quantify the amount of message per cell (proportional to the number of grains), and to look for hormone effects on oxytocin gene expression (Chung et al., 1991). First, they found that estrogen increased levels of oxytocin mRNA in certain anterior hypothalamic and preoptic nerve cells. Then, to study cells relevant to lordosis behavior, they back-filled paraventricular nucleus cell bodies using a retrograde tracer, fluorogold, applied to the spinal cord. Combining that with in situ hybridization, they found that high doses of estradiol were followed by significantly greater amounts of oxytocin mRNA in a subpopulation of these PVN neurons that project to the spinal cord (Chung et al., 1991, unpublished data). Their results are consistent with the existence of a functional estrogen response element (ERE) in the oxytocin gene promoter (Aden et al., 1992; Burbach et al., 1990; Mohr et al., 1988; Richard & Zingg, 1990). Also, we had shown estrogen binding in a relatively small number of oxytocin cells (Rhodes et al., 1981, 1982), which potentially could lead to Chung's result either through classical estrogen receptors (Warembourg & Poulain, 1991) or through the novel "estrogen receptor beta" (Kuiper et al., 1996).

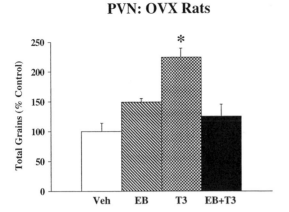

PVN: OVX Rats

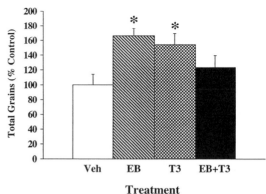

SON: OVX Rats

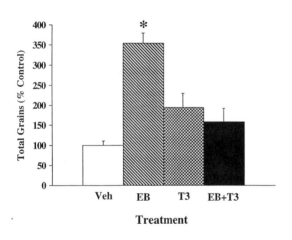

PVN: TX/OVX Rats

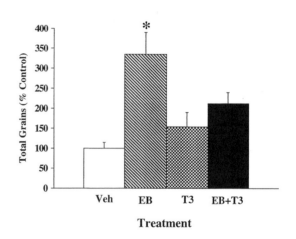

SON: TX/OVX Rats

Figure 10.4 Both in the hypothalamic paraventricular nucleus (*left,* PVN) and in the supraoptic nucleus (*right,* SON), the estrogen induction of oxytocin gene expression was larger in thyroidectomized or ovariectomized rats than that in simple ovex rats. Therefore, endogenous thyroid hormones were interfering with estrogen action. As well, the addition of thyroid hormone (T3) to the estrogen treatment (i.e., EB + T3) significantly reduced the effect of EB alone. Also see figure 7.11 for photomicrographs illustrating results from this experiment. (From Dellovade et al., 1998.)

(figure 10.5). By reverse transcriptase–polymerase chain reaction assay as well, estradiol treatment (but not progesterone) led to large increases in oxytocin receptor mRNA in the VMH (Breton & Zingg, 1997).

Therefore, estrogen effects on the ligand oxytocin and on its receptors, measured by molecular (Quiñones-Jenab et al., in press) and by electrophysiological (Kow et al., 1991) methods would *multiply* each other to achieve an even greater behavioral impact (Pfaff, 1988). The potential for an extended series of multiplicative mechanisms in the oxytocin neuronal system has been pointed out (Pfaff, 1988). Oxytocin predominantly excites other oxytocin neurons (Yamashita et al., 1987). Because estrogen turns on oxytocinergic neuronal electrical activity but not vasopressinergic cells (Akaishi & Sakuma, 1985), the hormone actually should set off a self-reexciting neuronal mechanism of considerable quantitative import. The theoretical possibilities are illustrated in figure 10.6 (Pfaff, 1988).

Multiplicative hormone effects are not limited to oxytocin (see figure 7.6). Massive estrogen effects on enkephalin gene expression (Lauber et al., 1990; Priest et al., 1996; Romano et al., 1988) would be multiplied by estrogen effects on gene expression for the delta opioid receptor, through which enkephalins act (Quiñones-Jenab et al., unpublished data). Likewise, long and strong estrogen treatment can increase gonadotropin-releasing hormone (GnRH) mRNA levels (Roberts et al., 1989; Rosie et al., 1990; Rothfeld et al., 1989) at the same time as estrogen stimulation of GnRH receptor gene expression has been reported (Quinones-Jenab; Jennes). All these systems (see figure 5.13) should serve to provide molecular mechanisms for stimulating estrogen-dependent reproductive behaviors. In turn, the behavioral action should be subject to the two qualifications already presented, which mirror each other. First, the oxytocin effect would facilitate social encounters by reducing the anxiety inherent in meeting the opposite gender (McCarthy et al., 1991, 1996). Second, indeed the oxytocin effect is limited to circumstances that provoke such anxiety (Fahrbach et al., 1986).

In chapter 8, we argued that the deepest biological roots of human sex drive depended on the forebrain mechanisms elucidated in this book and previously. Interestingly then, cellular and neurochemical features of these oxytocin

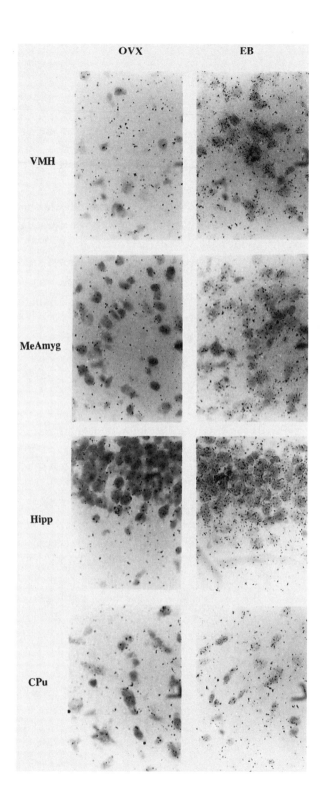

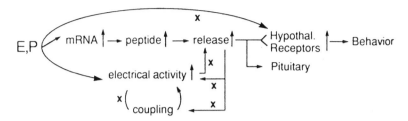

Figure 10.6 Original concept that sex steroid hormones can have *multiplicative* actions on neurons (Pfaff, 1988). This concept probably is exemplified in the most marked fashion by the oxytocin neuronal system. Not only does estradiol lead to increased gene expression for oxytocin MRNA in a subset of rat paraventricular hypothalamic neurons (Chung et al., 1991; Dellovade et al., 1998) but, importantly, estradiol leads to increased electrical activity in oxytocin neurons (Akaishi & Sakuma, 1985). Further, the novel findings of functional coupling among magnocellular neurons, discovered by Hatton, Theodosis, and Poulain, demonstrate a still greater opportunity for multiplicative actions of hormones. Finally, estrogens and progestins facilitate oxytocin receptors. (Additional references in Pfaff, 1988.)

◀ Figure 10.5   Estrogen-induced increases in oxytocin receptor messenger RNA in the ventromedial nucleus of the hypothalamus (VMH, *top*), the medial nucleus of the amygdala (MeAmyg), and the hippocampus (Hipp). A control region, the caudate-putamen (CPu, *bottom*) had low levels of expression and did not show an estrogen effect. (From Quiñones-Jenab et al., 1997.)

neurons seem to have been conserved in the human brain. Their anatomical organization is comparable in the human brain to that in nonhuman species (Sukhov et al., 1993), and the estrogen stimulation of oxytocin release remains in place in the human brain as well (Bossmar et al., 1995).

In summary, estrogen turns on a multiplicative oxytocinergic system that drives female reproductive behavior. Moreover (at least in mice), the oxytocin receptor system is strong in the female but not in the male (Chritin et al., 1996). In dramatic contrast to the positive estrogen effect, such severe stress as releases opioids can, under some circumstances, inhibit oxytocin neuronal activity (Russell et al., 1992; box 10.1). Naloxone, an opioid antagonist, impressively raised the electrical activity of oxytocin neurons, relieving them from their morphine-caused inhibition of electrical discharge, exemplifying how stress-caused opioid inputs could reduce oxytocin release (Bicknell et al., 1988). Under a variety of other circumstances, in rats mild stress can, instead, clearly cause oxytocin release. Overall, the pattern of results with oxytocin shows a pleasing isomorphism between molecular biology and reproductive behavior. We believe that oxytocin release actually serves to protect a broad variety of social responses from disruption due to mild stress.

C. COMPARISONS TO ANOTHER NEUROPEPTIDE: GONADOTROPIN-RELEASING HORMONE

GnRH neurons follow a developmental course the appreciation of which requires a good sense of humor. Instead of being born in the ependymal surfaces of the brain as are proper neurons, they are born in the olfactory placode and migrate up the nose and into the developing basal forebrain (see figure 6.17; Schwanzel-Fukuda & Pfaff, 1989). (The migration from nose to brain suggests that people who get a "nose job" will do so at their own risk!) More seriously, the cellular and molecular correlates of the GnRH neuronal migration have been explored (see figure 6.18).

Interruption of the GnRH neuronal migration in human males results in a loss of libido associated with Kallmann's syndrome (Schwanzel-Fukuda et al., 1989; see chapter 7). In experimental animals, during adulthood GnRH clearly stimulates mating behavior (Moss & Dudley, 1984; Moss & McCann, 1973; Pfaff, 1973). Sites of action include the hypothalamus and the midbrain central gray (figure 10.7; Sakuma & Pfaff, 1980d). These results cannot be "explained away" by GnRH actions on the pituitary, because they can be obtained in hypophysectomized female rats (Pfaff, 1973), and they are specific to GnRH (Moss & McCann, 1973). Blocking the GnRH receptor reduces mating behavior (Dudley et al., 1981). In fact, destroying the gene for GnRH disrupts normal estrus cycles and their associated behaviors, whereas replacement of GnRH by tissue grafts into the preoptic area of such females yields females whose lordosis behavior was comparable to that in normal animals (Gibson et al., 1987).

A sensible conclusion, therefore, is that long and strong estrogen treatments as promote sex behavior also can increase the mRNA for GnRH (Roberts et al., 1989; Rosie et al., 1990; Rothfeld et al., 1989). This effect is unlikely to be due to direct E action in the nuclei of GnRH neurons, as they have little or no classic estrogen receptor and virtually no high-affinity nuclear E binding (Shivers et al., 1983). Instead, many possible indirect routes of action are available, including estrogen effects on preoptic GABA neurons (Flugge et al., 1986), NPY neurons (Crowley & Kalra, 1987), neurotensin neurons (Ferris et al., 1984), and noradrenergic inputs (Herbison, 1997).

Because under behaviorally relevant conditions estrogen can increase GnRH mRNA, especially interesting is that gonadal steroids also can regulate GnRH receptors (Ban et al., 1990; Badr et al., 1988; Jennes et al., 1995). In the arcuate and ventromedial nuclei of the rat hypothalamus, GnRH mRNA levels are highest during the morning of proestrus (Jennes et al., 1996), perhaps reflecting an estrogenic stimulation of GnRH gene expression (Quiñones-Jenab et al., 1996). The multiplicative character of estrogenic effects on GnRH and its receptor would help the hormone's actions to reach a level of behavioral and endocrine significance.

Notable is that GnRH receptor requirements for ligands may differ slightly in the brain compared to the pituitary (Dudley et al., 1983; Sakuma & Pfaff, 1983; Zadina et al., 1981).

Therefore, in turning on the GnRH gene and its receptor (figure 10.8; see also figure 7.6) estrogen is upregulating a system that subsequently facilitates

Box 10.1
Theoretical summary of the opposing effects of sex hormones (see figure 10.6) and stress on oxytocin neurons

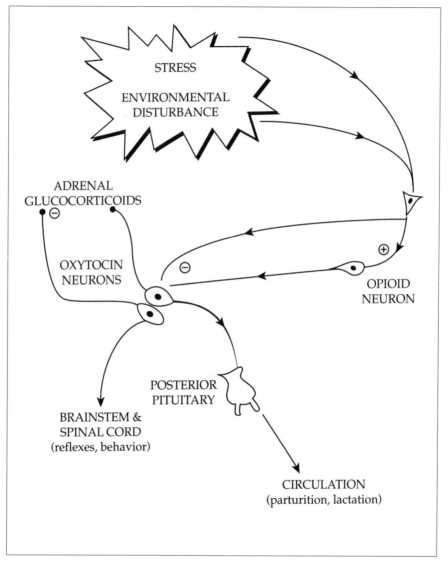

STRESS
ENVIRONMENTAL
DISTURBANCE

ADRENAL
GLUCOCORTICOIDS
⊖

OXYTOCIN
NEURONS
⊖

⊕

OPIOID
NEURON

POSTERIOR
PITUITARY

BRAINSTEM &
SPINAL CORD
(reflexes, behavior)

CIRCULATION
(parturition, lactation)

In figure 10.6 it was seen that estrogens can turn on a subset of oxytocin neurons, important at least as far as reproductive behavior is concerned. That is, estrogen increases gene expression in a specific subset of oxytocin neurons projecting to the brain and spinal cord, increases gene expression for the oxytocin receptor, and increases electrical activity in oxytocin neurons as would lead to a deposition of oxytocin into the synaptic cleft and its surround (Akaisha & Sakuma, 1985). The multiplicative character of estrogenic effects in the oxytocin system has been portrayed in figure 10.6. Here, from the work of John Russell and his colleagues in Edinburgh and Babringham (Douglas et al., 1997), we see that under some circumstances, stress reduces the functioning power of oxytocin neurons. Stress signals to neuroendocrine cells in the forebrain can be mediated, at the very least, by norepinephrine pathways arising from the hindbrain and, importantly, from opioid peptide neurons. This complex situation has been considered in a well-qualified manner by John Russell of the University of Edinburgh, and this brief summary comprises a digest and adaptation of his writings (Russell et al., 1995; Douglas et al., 1993). Briefly, environmental stress can reduce oxytocin secretion, can interfere with maternal behavior, and can slow parturition. Evidence for the important contribution of opioid peptide neurons comes from the demonstration that both the reduced secretion of oxytocin and consequent slowing of parturition are reversed by administration of the opioid antagonist naloxone. As powerful inhibitors as the opioid peptides might be, it is not a simple situation in which all inhibitory effects of environmental stress simply are mediated by endogenous opioids. Indeed, a marked "state dependence" is seen in the relationship between opioid peptides and oxytocin, one analogous to the state dependence of oxytocin effects on maternal behavior (Fahrbach et al., 1986). In virgin rats, the effect of naloxone, the opioid antagonist, on oxytocin secretion depends on the initial state of excitation in oxytocin neurons (Russell et al., 1995; Douglas et al., 1995).

Some indications suggest that oxytocin has suppressive effects on the hypothalamo-pituitary-adrenal axis, thus reducing adrenal glucocorticoids. This mechanism could be one by which oxytocin combats the disruptive effects of stress on reproductive and maternal behaviors.

In summary, maternal oxytocin is secreted in pulses from the posterior pituitary and is released synaptically in brain and spinal cord, consequent to synchronized burst-firing of oxytocin neurons (e.g., during parturition). Under some circumstances, environmental stress clearly reduces oxytocin secretion and slows parturition, whereas under other circumstances, stressors stimulate oxytocin secretion. In this latter case, oxytocin responses are restrained by endogenous opioids that act centrally to brake the excitation of oxytocin neurons. Thus, in the complex world of stress physiology, one signal comes through clearly: During parturition, the stress of environmental disturbance slows parturition by decreasing oxytocin secretion, and these effects are mediated by the inhibiting power of endogenous opiates.

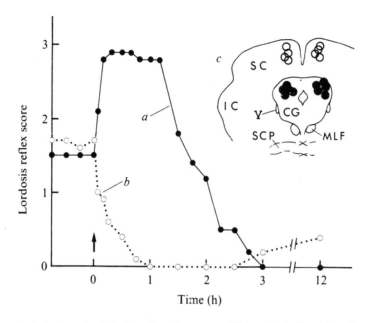

Figure 10.7   Direct microinjection of small amounts of GnRH (or LHRH) directly to the midbrain central gray (black circles, inset) significantly elevated the performance of lordosis (curve with black circles). If instead, an antibody against GnRH was microinjected into the central gray, lordosis behavior was reduced significantly (curve b, open circles). Applications at a control site in the superior colliculus (SC, open circles) were not effective. (From Sakuma & Pfaff, 1980d.)

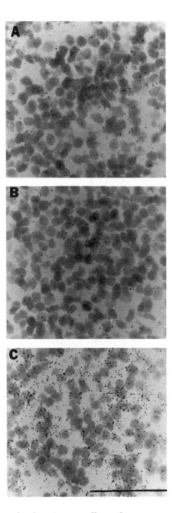

Figure 10.8   Photomicrographs showing an effect of estrogen on GnRH receptor messenger RNA, as demonstrated by in situ hybridization in pituitary gland tissue. The numbers of grains per cell were low in ovariectomized control females (*A*) and after only 12 hours of estrogen treatment (*B*). However; after 48 hours of estrogen treatment, (*C*), the numbers of cells labeled and the numbers of grains per cell were elevated significantly. (From Quiñones-Jenab et al., 1996).

mating. Even more than that, estrogen may be turning on a self-reexciting neuronal system, because GnRH neurons are connected to each other by synapses (reviewed by Ann Judith Silverman in Knobil & Neill, 1994) and by gap junctions (Jennes et al., 1998; Wetsel, 1995). Under specific conditions, activities of GnRH neurons are coordinated to form excitatory pulses (Knobil & Neill, 1994), perhaps because GnRH neurons have GnRH receptors (Krsmanovic et al., 1993). Mathematical modeling shows clearly that a population of GnRH neurons with excitatory connections can organize pulses of activity (Gordan et al., in press). Putting all this together reveals that a hormone-stimulated GnRH system should have the capacity powerfully to promote reproductive behavior, which in fact it does.

The behavioral roles for GnRH are even more amazing in view of the fact that the functions for which GnRH is justly famous are not behavioral at all. They are endocrine: GnRH was known for and named for its ability to release gonadotropins (luteinizing hormone and follicle-stimulating hormone) from the pituitary. What follows neatly is that the behavioral roles for GnRH join with the endocrine roles to direct a body-wide functional reproductive system.

The foregoing discussion leads to the principle that *through their actions in the brain, neuropeptides coordinate behavioral tendencies with their other actions throughout the body.* Their behavioral roles are congruent with their other physiological roles. Our GnRH action on mating behavior was the first demonstration of this principle, but oxytocin illustrates it just as well.

D. DIFFERENT NEUROANATOMICAL SYSTEMS FOR DIFFERENT DRIVES

Formerly, many thought that no real anatomical order could be discerned in the hypothalamus and basal forebrain because beautiful laminated structures, such as those apparent in thalamocortical systems and cerebellum, could not be seen there. However, new work with modern neuroanatomical techniques has revealed much more order than previously was expected. Cell groups in the hypothalamus and basal forebrain give rise to long axonal pathways that tend to be positioned according to the location of the cell bodies: dorsal cell groups with dorsal running axons, medial to medial, ventral to ventral, and so on (Conrad & Pfaff, 1976a,b; Krieger et al., 1979; Pfaff & Conrad, 1978). These tendencies toward "laminar flow" are not followed as rigidly as in neocortical systems but are illustrated easily both in a three-dimensional-style picture (see figure 5.11) and in cross-section (see figure 5.12).

Are these neuroanatomical differences associated with different functions? Yes. The first and most easily established functional circuit has been identified for female-typical lordosis behavior (chapter 6), controlled from the VMH through descending axons that run outside the medial forebrain bundle. In contrast, male mating behavior is controlled from neurons deep within the medial preoptic nucleus and diagonal bands of Broca through axons that run in the medial forebrain bundle. This findings seems constant across all vertebrate species (Kelley & Pfaff, 1978; Meisel & Sachs, 1994). Still another instinctive behavior, maternal behavior, depends on neurons in the lateral and dorsal part of the preoptic area, near the bed nucleus of the stria terminalis (Numan, 1994).

Further, functionally relevant anatomical distinctions have been discovered in other limbic-hypothalamic systems. Projections from different hippocampal regions through different septal regions to different hypothalamic zones have been mapped in a manner that reveals strong topographical organization (Risold & Swanson, 1996). The authors propose that different classes of these projections are related separately to agonistic, reproductive, and ingestive behaviors.

Thus, the current neuroanatomical picture is of limbic-hypothalamic systems that possess greater order than previously was suspected. Beyond that, we see that different drives have distinct anatomical representations among limbic and hypothalamic cell groups.

E. Summary

We have shown how different neuropeptides serve different behavioral roles related to broad social behavioral tendencies, operating through distinct neuroanatomical pathways. Hormone actions on the genes related to these neuropeptides can have a multiplicative character, affecting both the peptide ligand and its receptor. Some of these neuroendocrine peptide systems appear to have a self-reexciting character, well suited to the production of a large, behaviorally significant change. Neuropeptide effects depend precisely on the circumstances of behavioral assay; For example, oxytocin protects instinctive responses against mild stress and, correspondingly, depends on ambient stress level for its efficacy. Overall, an impressive degree of congruence exists between a neuropeptide's physiological and behavioral effects.

The following chapter illustrates still more global actions of sex hormones in the brain relevant to neuronal growth and behavioral capacities in aged individuals.

11

REPRODUCTIVE HORMONES, NEURONAL GROWTH, AND COGNITION

Something is taking its course.
You cried for night; it falls: now cry in darkness.

—Samuel Beckett, *Endgame,* 1958

Besides their prominent and well-documented effects on behaviors, sex hormones have actions in the brain that go well beyond any specific behavior and that might be important for the consideration of mental alterations during aging. The most frequently asked health questions about menopausal women taking estrogens center on their positive effects on cardiovascular health and on the maintenance of bone *versus* negative effects related to the risk of hormone-dependent cancerous growths. Another important consideration as to whether to take estrogens postmenopausally is the amelioration of hot flashes by estradiol. However, from the straight neurobiological point of view, the neuronal growth that follows estrogen treatment is, by far, the biggest story.

A. Estrogen-Stimulated Growth of Nerve Cells

1. Hypothalamic Neurons

The first hint that the very "power plant" of a nerve cell might be affected by estradiol came from striking alterations in the nucleolus and the nucleus and in hypothalamic cell bodies after estrogen treatment (figures 11.1 and 11.2). In January 1978, Dr. Rochelle Cohen was finishing her postdoctoral fellowship with the eminent cell biologist Professor Phillip Siekevitz. Having read about some of the biosynthetic and structural effects of steroid hormones outside the brain, the author was interested in neurobiological investigations of steroid hormone effects. Since I had injured my ankle, I hopped around the lab on one foot to perfuse brain tissue from ovariectomized female rats given either estradiol for 2 weeks or vehicle control treatment, in order properly to fix cells in the hypothalamus for Dr. Cohen to examine through the electron microscope. From her first publication in *Cell and Tissue Research* (Cohen & Pfaff, 1981) and extending for several years, this line of research turned out to be a rich source of new insights related to trophic actions of steroid hormones in the brain.

These first morphological structural effects of estrogen were revealed as a massive elaboration of the rough endoplasmic reticulum in hypothalamic nerve cells, in a region where neurons have estrogen receptors. We also saw a large increase in the number of prosecretory granules in the vicinity of the Golgi apparatus (figures 11.3 and 11.4). All these findings pointed to an increase in the biosynthetic activity of these hypothalamic nerve cells with estrogen receptors. Following those discoveries, Cohen and her student, Sookja Kim Chung, showed alterations on the surface of the nucleolus (a part of the "power plant" that makes ribosomal RNA) (see figure 11.1; Chung et al., 1984; Cohen et al., 1984). Cohen has reviewed these experiments (Cohen & Pfaff, 1992). Estrogen increased the appearance of ribosomal RNA's gene on the surface of the nucleolus, where ribosomal RNA would be synthesized. Later Dr. Kathryn J. Jones followed up the ribosomal RNA ideas by demonstrating not only the structural effects of estrogens acting in the nucleus (Jones et al., 1985) but

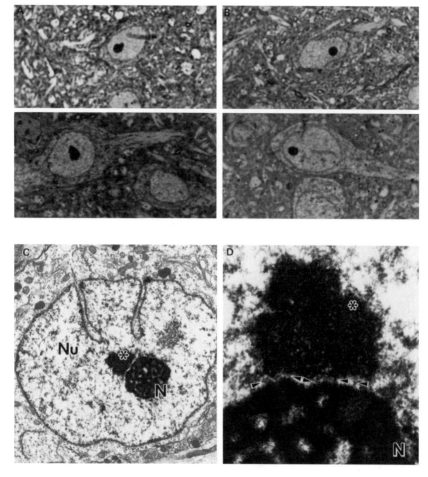

Figure 11.1 A "bump" appeared on the surface of the nucleolus of ventromedial hypo-thalamic cells with increased frequency in estrogen-treated female rats (Cohen et al., 1984). With the light microscope, instead of having a smooth surface (*B*), these cells had obvious ir-regular surface features (*A*). With higher magnification using the electron microscope (*C*), the surface feature (★) is seen to be prominent, electron-dense, and actually separated from the nucleolus (N) itself by a fine gap. In the nucleus (Nu) of this interesting ventromedial hy-pothalamic cell, at still higher magnification with the electron microscope (*D*), the material on the surface (★) is seen to penetrate the gap toward the nucleolus (N) with fine strands of electron-dense material (Cohen et al., 1984). Subsequent enzyme digestion studies (Chung et al., 1984) showed that this material on the surface and penetrating the gap is DNA. We concluded that these are genes for ribosomal RNA penetrating to the fibrillar centers of the nucleolus, thus to manufacture ribosomal RNA. This happens more frequently in estrogen ventromedial hypothalamic neurons and fits the data from the work of Dr. Kathryn J. Jones (see text and figures 11.5 and 11.6).

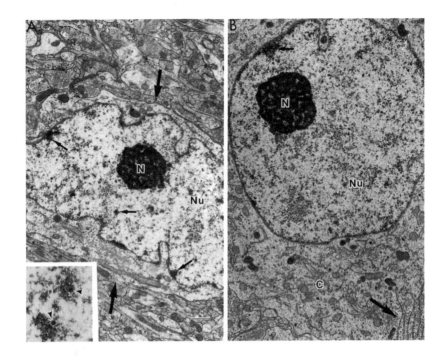

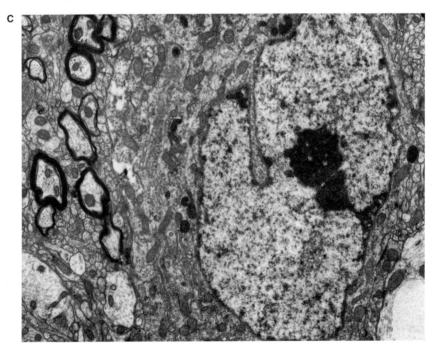

increased molecular hybridization products using radioactively labeled probes for in situ hybridization that would measure either newly synthesized or fully mature ribosomal RNA (Jones et al., 1986, 1990). Overall, Jones handily concluded that the molecular effects of estrogen on the generation of ribosomal RNA preceded the eventual structural alterations in hypothalamic neurons (figures 11.5 and 11.6).

A natural result of this increased capacity for synthetic activity in the power plant of the neuron is to increase the number of synapses. Sookja Kim Chung (Chung et al., 1988) was able to see an increase in the number of synapses from the hypothalamus after estrogen treatment, a finding reminiscent of the report by Carrer and Aoki (1982). This type of work was extended by Maya Frankfurt in Bruce McEwen's laboratory, showing an increased number of dendritic spines on hypothalamic neurons (Frankfurt, 1994; Gould et al., 1990).

In summary, this field of work has demonstrated that estrogen treatment can enhance the ability of hormone-sensitive hypothalamic neurons to produce proteins and to grow and that estrogen also increases the inputs and outputs of hypothalamic neurons to and from other cells. The full set of mechanisms for these changes have not been spelled out, but connections between steroid hormones and growth factors have been reported. For example, results of Dominique Toran-Allerand and Robert Gibbs in the central nervous system are consistent with those of Kenneth Korach who, in 1991, pointed out the effects of EGF on

Figure 11.2   Rapid ultrastructural alterations in ventromedial hypothalamic neurons (VMN) after only 2 hours of estradiol treatment. A comparison of an estradiol-treated female rat (B) with control ovariectomized rat (A) reveals that the nucleolus is bigger; the cell nucleus is bigger and has rounded up; fewer clumps of heterochromatin are seen (i.e., more frequent in A; see inset in A illustrating perichromatin granules), and the beginning of estrogen-stimulated stacking of rough endoplasmic reticulum (RER) is seen in the lower right corner of (B). (C, cytoplasm; N, nucleolus; Nu, nucleus.) (From K.J. Jones et al., 1985.) (C) Occasionally, in a hypothalamic neuron sampled from an estrogen-treated female rat, we could see a continuous path of electron-dense material from the surface of the nucleolus to the nuclear envelope. This event was seen rarely enough that we were never able to discern its functional significance but considered the possibility that it represented a type of exit route for newly synthesized ribosomal RNA.

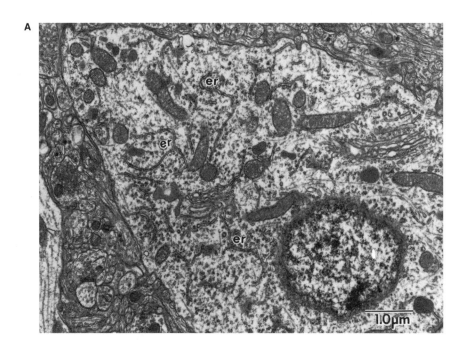

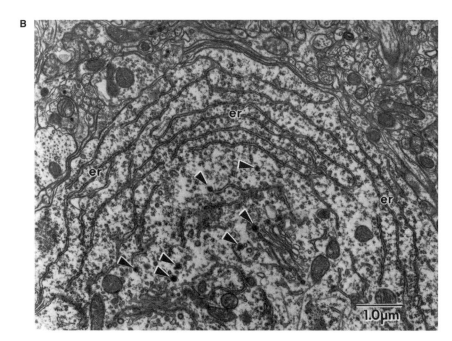

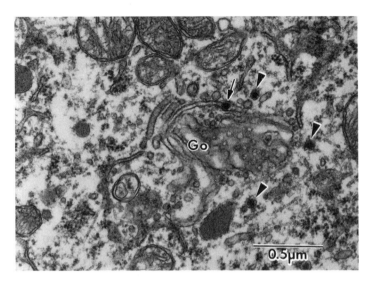

Figure 11.4   Electron micrograph at high magnification (see bar representing 0.5 μm) centering on the Golgi apparatus (Go) of a neuron in the ventrolateral subdivision of the ventromedial nucleus of the hypothalamus in an estrogen-treated rat. Animals treated with estrogen for 2 weeks demonstrated a large increase in the number of dense-cored vesicles (arrow and arrowheads) in the vicinity of the Golgi apparatus. Taking this finding together with the other molecular and morphological effects of estrogen on these ventromedial hypothalamic cells, we believe that the significant increase in the number of dense-cored vesicles reflects an estrogen-stimulated increase in the biosynthetic capacities of these cells. (Data from Cohen & Pfaff, 1981.)

◀ Figure 11.3   Estrogen stimulates the formation of rough endoplasmic reticulum (er) in ovariectomized female rats. (From Cohen & Pfaff, 1981.) (A) Ovariectomized control animals exhibit a relatively small amount of rough endoplasmic reticulum (er), not highly organized. (B) Animals treated with estradiol for 2 weeks exhibit a large amount of rough endoplasmic reticulum (er) arranged in parallel stacks. In both (A) and (B), electron micrographs were taken at a magnification of ×12,000. Estrogen-treated animals also exhibit many dense-cored vesicles (black arrowheads) that we interpret as prosecretory granules (see also figure 11.4).

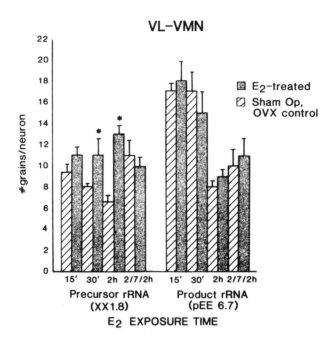

Figure 11.5   In situ hybridization was used with a probe directed against the external transcribed spacer of the rat ribosomal RNA nascent transcript, a region cleaved immediately after transcription and thus close to a measurement of transcription rate (Precursor rRNA). On a second set of slides, in situ hybridization was used with a probe against mature 18S rRNA (Product rRNA). In the ventromedial hypothalamus (VL-VMN) at very short times after the beginning of estrogen treatment, estradiol led to a significant increase in rRNA initial transcript levels. Mature rRNA levels went up later (see figure 11.6). Measurements in control regions showed no significant estrogen effects. (From Jones et al., 1990.)

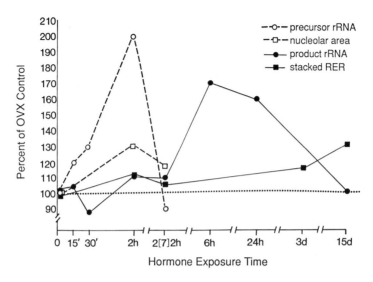

Figure 11.6   The most rapid effect of estradiol in Jones's histochemical and ultrastructural work was on the nascent transcript (Precursor) for rRNA. This was accompanied by changes in the nucleolus and nucleus of ventromedial hypothalamic cells and was followed by significant elevation of mature (Product) rRNA. The most striking morphological changes in the cytoplasm, including stacked rough endoplasmic reticulum (RER), followed on. All the morphological changes discovered by Cohen, Chung, and Jones bespoke a massive increase in operation of the "power plant" of the ventromedial hypothalamic neuron, indicating increased biosynthetic capacity. (From Jones & Pfaff, 1991.)

estrogen actions in the uterus. Recent reports have shown that estradiol can stimulate tyrosine phosphorylation of an insulinlike growth factor receptor (Richards et al., 1996). Conversely, neurotrophic factors can stimulate the expression of a sex hormone receptor in neurons (Al-Shamma & Arnold, 1996).

Even beyond the straightforward mechanisms spelled out in Potential Mechanisms, below, an entirely new possibility recently came up for helping to explain estrogen-stimulated neuronal growth. This new idea derives from the estrogen sensitivity of vascular endothelial growth factor (V-EGF; Hyder et al., 1996; McLaren et al., 1996; Shifren et al., 1996). The induction of V-EGF by estrogen is estrogen receptor–mediated, as a pure antiestrogen will block it (Chiappetta et al., 1997). Better vascularity could be part of the way E can help to protect against strokes (Paganini-Hill, 1995), β-amyloid toxicity (Behl et al., 1996; Goodman et al., 1996; Green et al., 1996), oxidative damage (Dluzen et al., 1996), and the consequences of penetrating brain injury (Garcia-Estrada et al., 1993). So, estrogenic effects on the cerebral vasculature could be important for hormonal facilitation of neuronal growth and repair.

Incidentally, an unexpected result of hypothalamic neuronal activity is that it actually maintains the health of certain neurons in the midbrain central gray (i.e., destruction of ventromedial hypothalamic cells can cause transsynaptic degeneration in the midbrain) (Chung et al., 1990). (For a 1997 overview, the picture of estrogen-stimulated neuronal growth is summarized in figure 11.7.)

2. NERVE CELLS OUTSIDE THE HYPOTHALAMUS

Examining possible implications of sex steroid effects on memory naturally necessitated examining the hippocampus, which revealed that estrogen can increase the number of dendritic spines in hippocampal pyramidal cells (Gould et al., 1990; Woolley et al., 1990; Woolley & McEwen, 1992). Other recent evidence as well shows that trophic actions of estrogens can be applied outside the hypothalamus. In female prairie voles, cell division in the ventricular and subventricular zones was facilitated by estrogen treatment, as shown by an increased number of BrdU-labeled cells (Smith et al., 1997).

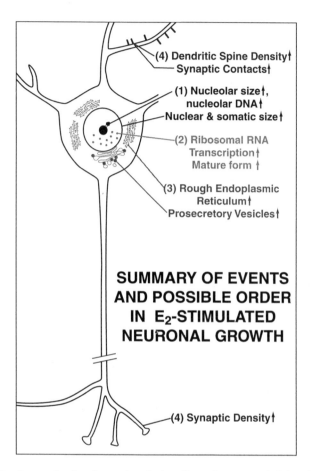

Figure 11.7   As a result of nuclear and nucleolar effects of estrogen administration, ribosomal RNA is transcribed at a greater rate, resulting in a significant increase in the amount of
mature rRNA. Morphologically, the rough endoplasmic reticulum burgeons, and prosecretory vesicles are increased in number. Presumably as a result of these developments in the
"power plant" of the neuron, dendritic spines and axonal terminals are increased in frequency.

The most amazing growth-related effect of estradiol occurs in a part of the brain never before associated with sex hormone action. In the cat brain, the nucleus retroambiguus is located in the caudal medulla and sends axons into the spinal cord, where they terminate among pelvic floor and other axial motoneurons (Vanderhorst & Holstege, 1997). Most surprising to see is that the density of axonal terminations among their target motoneuronal cell groups from this descending system was much greater in the presence of high levels of estrogen (figure 11.8; Vanderhorst & Holstege, 1997). As a neuroanatomical control for specificity of the hormone effect, the rubrospinal pathway displayed no differences. Labeled growth cones were seen in the descending retroambiguus pathways of estrous (but not nonestrous) cats. This article was the first demonstration of trophic actions of estrogen in a brainstem system descending to the spinal cord.

B. HORMONES AND NEURONAL REPAIR

Steroid sex hormones are not limited to straightforward neuronal growth effects; they also can help with neuronal repair (Baulieu, 1996). Understanding the effects of progesterone metabolites in neuronal repair importantly requires the knowledge that glial cells, oligodendrocytes in culture, can manufacture myelin basic protein (Jung-Testas et al., 1989, 1991) and that as a component of neuronal repair, myelin biogenesis has been analyzed extensively (Barry et al., 1996; Hardy & Friedrich, 1996).

Also interesting is that certain progesterone metabolites actually can be synthesized in the brain within glial cells (Schumacher & Baulieu, 1995). For example, the biosynthesis of pregnenolone was demonstrated by incubating rat glial cells with a labeled precursor of cholesterol and the subsequent isolation of labeled pregnenolone (Jung-Testas et al., 1989). In turn, pregnenolone can be converted to progesterone, which is metabolized by 5α-reductase and 3α-hydroxysteroid oxidoreductase to its reduced metabolites (Schumacher & Baulieu, 1995). Such neurosteroids are active in neuronal repair.

A major feature of neuronal repair is the replacement of myelin in wounded nerve. In view of the foregoing facts generated in their laboratory and

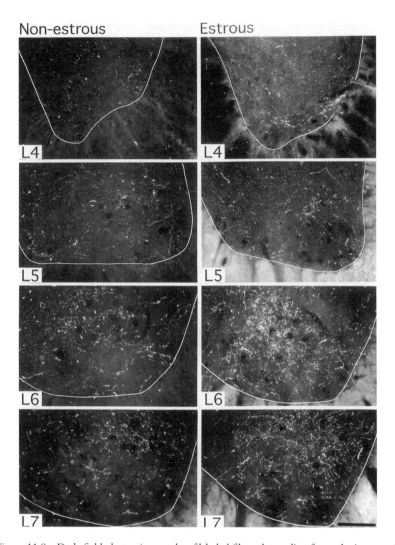

Figure 11.8   Dark-field photomicrographs of labeled fibers descending from a brainstem cell group, the nucleus retroambiguus, to the lumbar spinal cord. As shown by the comparison between an estrous animal (*right*) and a nonestrous animal (*left*), estrogen induced axonal outgrowth in this pathway descending from the brainstem to the spinal cord. (From Vanderhorst & Holstege, 1997.)

of the history of work on hormone metabolism in the brain, Schumacher and Baulieu hypothesized that progesterone metabolites produced by glial cells would assist in the process of remyelination. To test this hypothesis, they made cryolesions of the sciatic nerve in male mice, because these axons are known to be able to regenerate and become myelinated. Blocking either the local synthesis or the receptor-mediated action of progesterone impaired remyelination (Koenig et al., 1995). Conversely, administration of progesterone to the lesion site increased the extent of myelin sheath formation. Also, myelination of axons was increased when progesterone was added to cultures of rat dorsal root ganglia (Koenig et al., 1995). As well, progesterone administration reduces the extent of neuronal damage after middle cerebral artery occlusion (Jiang et al., 1996). Thus, progesterone metabolites may assist in neuronal repair.

Finally we expect that estrogen treatment also could protect against toxicological insults to nerve cells (e.g., damage by glutamate toxicity) (Singer et al., 1996). More generally, steroid sex hormones now are known not to be limited in their cerebral functions to reproductive neuroendocrine phenomena and reproductive behaviors and drives but also promote neuronal growth (see Estrogen-Stimulated Growth of Nerve Cells) and repair.

C. Implications for Cognitive Functions

Especially with the "baby-boomer" generation reaching age 50, a large part of our population not only is concerned with the normal decline in memory functions during normal aging but is even more afraid of memory loss as a result of Alzheimer's disease. Estrogens can ameliorate this problem, essentially delaying the loss of function, and the experimental evidence comes from work with both humans and animals.

1. Evidence from Humans

At Rockefeller University in the 1980s, a young doctor named Howard Fillit began a pilot study to explore possible effects of estrogen on memory loss in the aged. Some of the women in his sample appeared to show marked gains in their cognitive skills. A recent population study provided additional support for the possible amelioration of Alzheimer's symptoms by estrogen treatment. Estrogen replacement therapy recipients had only 0.46 the risk for Alzheimer's disease as compared to nonuser controls (Kawas et al., 1997)

Professor Barbara Sherwin, at McGill University in Montreal, has turned this question into a clear conclusion, as follows: First, during a long series of tests in 19 women who required hysterectomy and bilateral oophorectomy, estrogen therapy prevented a significant decrease in memory recall of paired-associate learning items (Phillips & Sherwin, 1992a). The estrogen effect on memory helps to explain variations across the menstrual cycle and can be distinguished from potential progesterone effects: Plasma progesterone in the luteal phase of the cycle was correlated with decreased visual memory (Phillips & Sherwin, 1992b). In young women whose ovarian hormones were reduced by long-term treatment with a gonadotropin–releasing hormone agonist, estrogen treatment reversed memory deficits that were apparent in the group receiving only placebo after agonist-induced hypoestrogenism (Sherwin & Tulando, 1996). Likewise, in a group of healthy postmenopausal women, the scores of subjects taking estrogen were significantly higher on tests of immediate and delayed paragraph recall, as compared to scores of nonusers. No differences were apparent on other tests of cognition, including spatial memory (Kampen & Sherwin, 1994).

In other laboratories as well, tests showed that memory and attention can be improved by estrogen treatment in postmenopausal women, with an emphasis on better maintenance of verbal memory performance as opposed to spatial functions (Ross, 1997). Professor Doreen Kimura's sample of postmenopausal women also had better scores on a battery of cognitive functions if they were on estrogen replacement therapy (Kimura, 1995).

The estrogen advantage is not necessarily restricted to women. In healthy young men, two measures of visual memory were higher in those subjects with high levels of circulating estradiol than with those with low levels (Kampen & Sherwin, 1996).

Overall, these findings over the last several years have provided substantial support for the hypothesis that estrogens can maintain short- and long-term verbal memory during aging, even under circumstances not exhibiting positive effects on visuospatial memory (Sherwin, 1994). Such findings are likely to have implications for the amelioration of symptoms in Alzheimer's disease. Dr. Sally Schumacher, at Bowman Gray School of Medicine in North Carolina, reported preliminary findings at a scientific meeting in Osaka, Japan, that a mixture of estrogens (Premarin) can at least delay the dementia of Alzheimer's disease. Dr. Stanley Birge, at Washington University School of Medicine in St. Louis, MO, has reviewed population studies indicating that women who took estrogen after menopause have a reduced incidence of Alzheimer's disease (Birge, June 1997, J. Amer. Geriatrics Society). Consistent with the animal brain data, reviewed below, therefore, estrogens protect against disease- or drug-induced loss of certain types of memory and against loss of function during normal aging.

2. ANIMAL LEARNING EXPERIMENTS

The regulation of learning and memory in female rats as they might be altered by estrogen has been analyzed thoroughly by Gary Dohanich and his colleagues at Tulane University in New Orleans. In an eight-arm radial maze, 30 days of estrogen pretreatment significantly improved memory compared to memory in females treated with the control substance cholesterol (Dohanich et al., 1997). Daniel and Dohanich (1997) reported that females receiving estrogen prior to training, during training, or at both periods performed better in the radial arm maze than did control females. They found also that estrogen treatment could reverse the impairments of memory caused by the cholinergic (muscarinic) antagonist scopolamine (Fader et al., 1997). Dohanich and his colleagues sharply distinguished these positive effects of estrogen from its lack of help in highly spatial tasks. Their results form a beautiful parallel with the data from human observations.

Independently, Professor Robert Gibbs et al. (1997) at the University of Pittsburgh also examined the possible effects of estrogen replacement on memory impairments induced by lorazepam or scopolamine. In a passive avoidance task, estrogen significantly attenuated the damaging effects of lorazepam on memory but had no effects if scopolamine were used as the amnestic agent.

Professor Victoria Luine (1997), at Hunter College in New York, also was able to see estrogen-enhanced performance in the eight-arm radial maze reflected, for example, in a smaller number of errors when delays of up to 4 hours were introduced. To test the generality of this type of cognitive enhancement, Richards et al., (1997) used an object recognition task in which unfamiliar objects were introduced for the measurement of investigation time. Long-term estrogen treatment was required for improved object recognition ability.

In summary, several laboratories have reported positive effects of estrogen on memory in ovariectomized female rats. None of them are simply thinking of estradiol as a "smart pill." Instead, limitations apply as to the duration of estrogen exposure, the nature of the task employed, and the amnestic challenge against which estrogen improvement militates.

3. POTENTIAL MECHANISMS

The primary mechanisms underlying the protective effects of estrogens on cognitive function are likely to be the first ones discovered: the growth-related actions of estrogen on the "power plant" of the neuron (reviewed in Estrogen-Stimulated Growth of Nerve Cells). After all, if all the protein synthetic machinery of a neuron (including both the nucleus and the cytoplasm) is "revved up" (Chung et al., 1984; Cohen & Pfaff, 1981; Jones et al., 1985, 1990), what follows is that dendrites can grow, axons can grow, synapses can be formed, and the memory functions that depend on those synapses can flourish.

One component of the growth cone in actively growing axons is the phosphoprotein growth-associated protein GAP-43. In our laboratory, Lustig et al. (1991) found 48% to 74% increases in the messenger RNA (mRNA) for GAP-43 in the ventromedial hypothalamus within 2 hours of estrogen treatment, an effect likely to represent a stimulation of GAP-43 gene transcription by estrogen. More recently, Singer and Dorsa (Singer et al., 1996) also noted estrogenic stimulation of GAP-43 mRNA in the preoptic area and found that an age-related decline could be reversed by estrogen treatment. Clearly, such estrogenic actions as this could contribute to the behavioral phenomena previously noted.

With respect to a different type of mechanism, Professor Victoria Luine has shown that estrogen administration to ovariectomized female rats can increase the levels of the enzyme that produces the transmitter acetylcholine (ACh), a potentially important finding, as Alzheimer's disease patients suffer a massive loss of ACh neurons in their basal forebrains. The complex of changes in cholinergic neuronal molecular mechanisms and in the mRNAs for nerve growth factor receptors may contribute to the types of neurochemical and behavioral results reported above (Gibbs et al., 1997; McMillan et al., 1996).

Still another potential mechanism concerns the receptor for the excitatory transmitterlike substance NMDA. Professor John Morrison, from Mt. Sinai School of Medicine, and Dr. Nancy Weiland have found 30% more of it in certain hippocampal neurons only in those female rats treated with estrogen. Finally, a Columbia University researcher who early had reported sprouting of cell processes in response to hormonal treatment now has shown a degree of cooperation between estrogens and nerve growth factor, each possibly amplifying the other's effects on nerve cell growth (Toran-Allerand et al., 1983). Notable also are the protective effects of estrogens (see Hypothalamic Neurons). Thus, ample morphological, neurochemical, and molecular evidence already is in place to begin providing theoretical explanations of memory enhancement due to estrogen treatment, and this dynamic field is growing rapidly.

D. HORMONE EFFECTS ON MOOD AND ANXIETY

Both estrogens and progestins have effects on mood and anxiety in women. Results from the observations of Dr. Uriel Halbreich regarding progesterone and from Dr. David Rubinow regarding estrogens have been reviewed (American Psychiatric Association Press, series edited by U. Halbreich). Typically, hypogonadal subjects have decreased libido, sexual function, and vigor but also have mood changes (Schmidt et al., 1997)

Changes during the menstrual cycle have suggested that "negative moods" would not be related to estrogens at all but definitely would depend on changes in progesterone levels (Schechter et al., 1996; see also Schechter et al., 1989).

The role of estrogens in significantly improving mood (i.e., combating depression) has been documented clearly during hormone replacement therapies (Rubinow & Schmidt, 1996; Stahl, 1996; see also Aylward, 1976; Daly et al., 1993; Limouzin-Lamothe et al., 1994; Michael et al., 1970). Interestingly, this finding is not necessarily limited by cultures, as Chinese women with postpartum depression were found to have decreased levels of estradiol in the blood (Lu et al. 1996). The power of estrogen in fighting depression is robust, such that oral estrogen can stem the onset of postpartum affective disorder in women with a history of puerperal major depression (Sichel et al., 1995). A caveat is in order here: The effects of estrogen on mood can be context-dependent and may vary according to the individual. For example, in 10 women with severe premenstrual mood changes, estrogen administration was associated with a recurrence of symptoms (Schmidt et al., 1998).

In dramatic contrast, high levels of progesterone (as during the late luteal phase of the menstrual cycle) in some women can be associated with negative changes in mood 4 to 6 days later (Halbreich et al., 1996). Negative moods would include sadness, tearfulness, irritability, depression, anxiety, or social withdrawal, and might be especially severe in individuals known to have a susceptibility to depression.

Metabolites of progesterone are an entirely different story. Those metabolites reduced in ring A at the fourth and fifth carbons are famous in their roles as anxiety reducers (anxiolytics). This mood effect has been documented in humans as well as in animals (Holzbauer, 1971; Majewska et al., 1986; Freeman et al., 1993; Picazo & Fernandes-Guasti, 1995; Bitran et al., 1991, 1993; Fernandes-Guasti, 1992; Rodriguez-Sierra et al., 1984; Weiland et al., 1991). It depends on the ability of reduced progesterone metabolites to enhance the

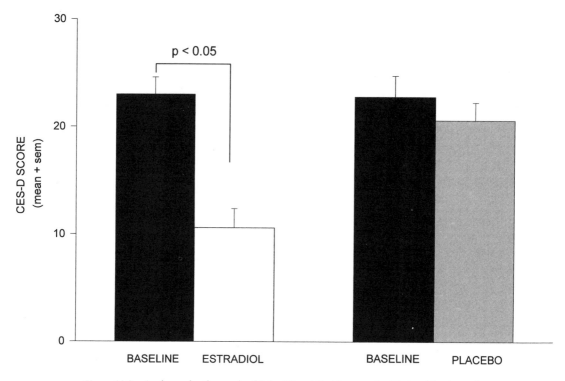

Figure 11.9 As shown by the work of Schmidt and Rubinow at the National Institutes for Mental Health (illustrated in this histogram) estrogens can heighten mood in women. Here, the authors report the effect of estrogen replacement on depression ratings in women with perimenopausal depression. A significant *reduction* in depression scores [Center for Epidemiologic Studies–Depression (CES-D) scale] was observed in 18 women who had received 3 weeks of estradiol treatment but not in 16 women who had received 3 weeks of placebo. Schmidt and Rubinow also noted that the effects of hormones on mood can be context-dependent and vary with the individual (Schmidt et al., 1998).

activity of the benzodiazepine-sensitive portion of the GABA-A receptor and thus to calm the recipient.

In summary, estrogens can heighten mood, whereas progesterone administration can be followed by depression, especially if accompanied by rapidly declining estrogen levels (figure 11.9). Mechanisms still are being worked out. Even though progesterone metabolites are relatively well understood as they enhance GABA receptor function, progesterone itself needs more work. Progesterone administration to female rabbits depressed midbrain reticular and cortical electrical activity (Kawakami & Sawyer, 1959). That result indeed could predict depressive mood effects, but more electrophysiology and, especially, more analysis of the genes turned on by progesterone in the brain is needed and is being conducted (Krebs et al., 1997).

Estrogenic mechanisms are so strong as to represent a form of "psychoprotection" (Fink, 1995). Apparently, estrogenic stimulation of a subset of serotonin receptors (5-HT-2A receptors) represents part of the mechanism (Fink et al., 1996), and estradiol also increases serotonin transporter mRNA levels in female rat brain (McQueen et al., 1997). Precisely how these molecular changes in monoamine neurochemistry cause locomotor and other muscular changes in female rodents and mood changes in women remains to be proved.

E. SUMMARY

Beyond the specific instinctive behaviors and motivational states the analysis of which yielded lawful results in molecular, neural, and biological terms, sex hormones also have much more global effects in brain tissue. They influence the "power plants" of neurons so as to produce growth of various sorts, and these very trophic actions might be at the base of cognitive enhancements reported for animals and humans. Moreover, the mood-related effects of estrogens and progestins in women are recognized widely. All these medically significant actions of sex hormones in the brain render the discovery of new tissue-selective estrogens and progestins fairly compelling, especially for their helpful effects during aging.

12

REFLECTION

During all of the twentieth century, neurobiologists have confronted the daunting complexity of the mammalian central nervous system. With the tremendous numbers of neurons involved and even larger numbers of connections between them, how can we make sense of higher brain function? How can we explain why a particular stimulus evokes a particular behavioral response at one time and not at another?

In this book, chapters 4 through 9 recount how a specific type of drive arises and leads to a specific behavior. The mechanism starts with the consequences of hormone receptor occupation in particular neurons, moves on to elevated expression of specific genes in those neurons, and subsequently uses altered hypothalamic outputs through a well-documented neuronal circuit to cause reproductive behavior. Thus, a mammalian behavior is determined by identified genes working in defined neuronal groups, affecting the behavioral response to a specific social stimulus. Beyond this focused demonstration, a reflection upon broader aspects of hormone actions in brain tissue would be timely.

FROM GENERAL INFLUENCES TO SPECIFIC RESULTS

Some of the results presented here imply the possibility for certain very general influences on the nervous system to yield specific behavioral results. Estrogens appear to act on ascending reticular activating systems, yielding an animal that is very active, alert, and muscularly taut. We notice a female whose overall demeanor suggests a condition of heightened arousal, broadly defined. Likewise, estrogens turning on the gene for the opioid peptide enkephalin apparently cause a state of partial analgesia in the female, in which strong cutaneous and visceral stimuli from the male can be tolerated (Bodnar et al., 1999). Yet, the most striking and obvious result of estrogenic action on the brain of the female rodent is the very specific sexual behavior of lordosis.

How is this so? The broad state of arousal is shown to lead to a series of courtship behaviors that prime lordosis behavior circuitry (see chapter 6). Then, the state of partial analgesia permits the lower brainstem and spinal cord to execute lordosis behavior, given proper stimulation from the male. Thus, even with particular genes (see chapter 7) and hypothalamic neurons (see chapter 6) powerfully brought into play, an important part of the specificity of neural control over this behavior lies in the stimulus itself.

From Specific to General

In chapters 10 and 11, on the other hand, particular effects of peptide hormones or steroids lead to consequences that are fairly general in their import. Oxytocin not only fosters lordosis behavior, working through its receptors in hypothalamic neurons, but encourages numerous behaviors that have as their underlying theme a high degree of affiliation with other animals. Another neuropeptide, gonadotropin-releasing hormone, promotes lordosis behavior indeed but also triggers a large number of changes (indirectly) throughout the body of the female. Finally, in chapter 11, we saw that estrogens, by encouraging neuronal growth, could influence broadly varied cognitive capacities and also could affect mood.

Questions for the Future

Where is this field of work going? The effort to understand neural and molecular mechanisms in the brain important for controlling behavior clearly represents "a now and future field." This, despite the fact that some of the most power-ful leaders of medical research in the United States have erred badly in assum-ing that research trying to explain behavior simply is not very good. Admittedly in the past, psychologists attempting to tackle the most complex problems of thought, feeling, and language perhaps sometimes have bitten off more than they could chew. However, many neurobiologists are ex–physics students with a strong inclination to strive for universal lawfulness and precise quantification. Our own trick has been to choose a simple enough behavioral problem that lawful solutions were achievable and to avail ourselves of all the tools of mo-lecular endocrinology, so that mechanisms could be laid bare. Getting the cir-cuit for a behavior has provided concrete proof that mechanisms of behavior, even for higher animals, now can be understood.

GENES

The human genome project and (following on) the mouse genome project are likely to be completed ahead of schedule and under budget. Consequently, the DNA revolution, spawned by the discovery by Watson and Crick (1953; Crick, 1962) and culminating in functional genomics, will stimulate a tremendous amount of work in neurobiology, just as it has done in other areas of medical re-search. Good choices of mammalian behaviors to study will allow us to demon-strate the codetermination of a wide range of behaviors by gene expression, internal physiological signals, and environmental stimuli. Our field of biology has established (see chapter 7) that an array of hormone-influenced genes partic-ipate both directly and indirectly in the facilitation of mating behavior. How-ever, the complexity of certain indirect effects (Pfaff, 1997) defies oversimplified thinking in the area of gene-behavior relationships. Recent findings using fruit flies (Drosophila) occasionally have led to the expectation, especially among non-scientists, of "one gene–one behavior" causal relationships. In higher organisms, this notion clearly will not be true. Instead, we will discover, step by step, how individual gene products are woven into neurobehavioral mechanisms, in some cases as a result of developmental effects and in other cases during adulthood.

In the nervous system, as in other organs, fruitful research will connect specific disease manifestations (Imura, 1997) with genetic disorders of steroid hormone receptors or metabolism (e.g., Shizuta et al., 1995). Peptide hormones produced by neurons present such opportunities, as well. For example, oxytocin and vasopressin have been cloned by Professor Dietmar Richter and his colleagues at the University of Hamburg (Ivell & Richter, 1984; Land et al., 1982; Mohr et al., 1995). The diabetes insipidus resulting from a mutation in the vasopressin gene (Schmale & Richter, 1984) is associated with defective transport of the mutant protein (Olias et al., 1996), an interesting defect in neurons known for targeted extrasomatic messenger RNAs (Kindler et al., 1997).

Especially during the ascendance of molecular genetics, studies of hormone effects on the brain will continue to be popular, because they allow all the tools of experimental endocrinology and molecular endocrinology to be applied to the questions of neurobiology. Most prominently, both in academic neuroendocrinology and in the public consciousness, sex differences have received a lot of attention.

SEX DIFFERENCES

Unfortunately, in recent American and European history, questions about sex differences became as "hot" politically as they were scientifically. Narrow-minded polemicists often heard many years ago during the first wave of American feminism simply denied sex differences in brain and behavior. They were mistaken. On the other hand, sex differences definitely are limited. In terms of neural mechanisms, the farther away the considered system is from actual reproductive neuroendocrine cells, the less statistically reliable and more functionally obscure tend to be the sex differences reported. Regarding human behavior, moods are demonstrably sensitive to hormones in some individuals, whereas sex differences in cognitive performance are difficult to demonstrate. Where human cognitive sex differences have been reported, what must be admitted, at least, is that eliminating potential social causes from consideration is almost impossible. In a population wherein girls do not do as well at mathematics as do boys, ruling out subtle influences from mathematics teachers who themselves have outdated attitudes is very difficult.

Therefore, acknowledging and even celebrating sex differences in the central nervous system is timely, but we must avoid overdrawing or overgeneralizing from the solid neuroendocrine differences that are proved. Mechanisms of hypothalamic and spinal cord differentiation still are under active investigation, and their implications for the patterning of social behavior remain relatively unexplored.

PROTEIN CHEMISTRY

Even with the increasingly sophisticated tools of neuroanatomy and electrophysiology, part of the driving force for twenty-first century neurobiological research is likely to come from protein chemistry and biophysics. For example, pharmacological and genetic manipulations of the functions of receptors on the nerve cell surface and of signaling systems in the cytoplasm and nucleus will allow us to add detail to every mechanism spelled out with established cell biological and electrophysiological techniques.

BEHAVIOR

The "bottom line" for all brain research will continue to be the understanding of behavior. Already, thorough dissections of mechanisms for learning and memory have incorporated molecular findings and represent a dynamic field in neurophysiology (Abel et al., 1998; Alberini & Kandel, 1995; Bailey et al., 1996). In the work presented in this book, increasingly detailed physiological and molecular analyses have always dictated sophisticated behavioral measurement for full comprehension of their central nervous system expression. Following logically is that behavioral neuroscience for its own sake will have to grow apace with molecular neurobiology.

PRIMITIVE FEELINGS IN HUMANS

Modern neurobiological perspectives allow for an understanding of biological desires in human beings, freed from a burden of guilt. Old-fashioned applications of traditional religious strictures often counterposed libidinal desires with "correct," moral behavior. From the point of view of well-regulated neural controls over biologically adaptive instinctive behaviors, that type of philosophy led to a set of prohibitions that, in any case, often were not followed but sometimes did cause psychological or social pathology. Instead, in projecting from discoveries about hormone actions on brain and behavior in animals, we can appreciate more fully how libidinal desires serve the human species well: Apollonian served by Dionysian, as well as the reverse. The relations of primitive human feelings to more elevated concerns, such as the formation of social values, will occupy philosophers as frequently as neural and behavioral biologists.

Overall, the orchestration of biological mechanisms centered around sex and social behaviors is more intricate than might have been imagined. Inevitably, the discoveries of neuroendocrinology in its molecular and behavioral aspects will be applied to human ills (real and imagined). The most obvious outlet from this new knowledge will be toward the neuropharmacology intended to deal with social and psychological problems connected with instinctive behaviors (aggression, sex, eating, sleeping, etc.) and mood disorders. As well, understanding the biological structure of neuronal mechanisms underlying these functions will pave the way for more informed and sensitive behavioral therapies.

REFERENCES

Abel, T., Martin, K., Bartsch, D., Kandel, E. Memory suppressor genes: Inhibitory constraints on the storage of long-term memory. *Science* 279:338-341, 1998

Acher, R. Neurohypophysial peptide systems: Processing machinery, hydroosmotic regulation, adaptation and evolution. *Regul. Pept.* 45:1–13, 1993

Aden, R.A.H., Lopes da Silva, S.F., Rigter, J.J.C.H., Burbach, J.P.H. Characterization of hormone response elements in rat oxytocin promoter. *J. Soc. Neurosci.* 18(1):241, 1992

Akaishi, T., Sakuma, Y. *J. Physiol. (Lond.)* 372:207–220, 1986

Akaishi, T., Sakuma, Y. Oestrogen excites oxytocinergic but not vasopressinergic cells in the paraventricular nucleus of the female rat. *Brain Res.* 335:302–305, 1985

Alberini, C.M., Kandel, E.R., et al. A molecular switch for the consolidation of long-term memory: cAMP-inducible gene expression. *Ann. N.Y. Acad. Sci.* 758:261–286, 1995

Alexander, G., Swerdloff, R., Wang, C., et al. Androgen-behavior correlations in hypogonadal men and eugonadal men. *Horm. Behav.* 31:110–119, 1997

Al-Shamma, H., Arnold, A. Brain-derived neurotrophic factor regulates expression of androgen receptors in perineal motoneurons. *Proc. Natl. Acad. Sci. U.S.A.* 1996

Andén, N.E., Dahlström, A., Fuxe, K., et al. Ascending noradrenaline neurons from the pons and the medulla oblongata. *Experiencea* 22:44–45, 1966

Andersson, S., Russell, D.W., Wilson, J.D. 17β-Hydroxysteroid dehydrogenase-3 deficiency. *Trends Endocrinol. Metab.* 7:121–126, 1996

Appelberg, B., Emonet-Denand, F. Motor units of the first superficial lumbrical muscle of the cat. *J. Neurophysiol.* 30:154–160, 1967

Arnold, A., Wade, J., Grisham, W., et al. Sexual differentiation of the brain in songbirds. *Dev. Neurosci.* 18:124–136, 1996

Aston-Jones, G., Rajkowski, J., Kubiak, P., et al. Role of the locus coeruleus in emotional activation. *Prog. Brain Res.* 107:379–402, 1996

Attardi, B. Facilitation and inhibition of the estrogen-induced luteinizing hormone surge in the rat by progesterone: Effects on cytoplasmic and nuclear estrogen receptors in the hypothalamus-preoptic area, pituitary, and uterus. *Endocrinology* 108:1487–1496, 1981

Attardi, B., Geller, L.N., Ohno, S. Androgen and estrogen receptors in brain cytosol from male, female and testicular feminized (Tfm/y hermaphrodite) mice. *Endocrinology* 98:864, 1976

Attardi, B., Klatt, B., Hoffman, G.E., Smith, M.S. Facilitation or inhibition of the estradiol-induced gonadotropin surge in the immature rat by progesterone: Regulation of GnRH and LH messenger RNAs and activation of GnRH neurons. *J. Neuroendocrinol.* 9:589–599, 1997

Attardi, B., Ohno, S. Physical properties of androgen receptors in brain cystosol from normal and testicular feminized (Tfm/Y hermaphrodite) mice. *Endocrinology* 103:760–770, 1978

Axelson, J.F., Sawin, C. Effects of voluntary and forced exercise on lordosis behavior in female rats. *Horm. Behav.* 21:384–392, 1987.

Aylward, M. Estrogens: Plasma tryptophan levels in perimenopausal patients. In S. Campbell (Ed.), *The management of the menopause and post-menopausal years.* Dallas: University Park Press, 1976:135–147

Badr, M., Marchetti, B., Pelletier, G. *Peptides* 9:441–442, 1988

Badr, M., Pelletier, G. *Synapse* 1:567–571, 1987

Bailey, C.H., Bartsch, D., Kandel, E.R. Toward a molecular definition of long-term memory storage. *Proc. Natl. Acad. Sci. U.S.A.* 93:13445–13452, 1996

Bakkum, B.W., Pfaff, D.W., Cohen, R.S. Lordosis-associated synaptic plasticity in the ventromedial hypothalamus (VMH) [abstract 80.4]. *J. Soc. Neurosci.* 21:188, 1995

Bale, T., Dorsa, D. Cloning: Novel promoter sequence, and estrogen regulation of a rat oxytocin receptor gene. *Endocrinology* 138:1151–1158, 1997

Bale, T.L., Dorsa, D.M. Sex differences in and effects of estrogen on oxytocin receptor mRNA expression in the ventromedial hypothalamus. *Endocrinology* 136:27–32, 1995

Bale, T.L., Dorsa, D.M., Johnston, C.A. Oxytocin receptor mRNA in the ventromedial hypothalamus during estrous cycle. *J. Neurosci.* 15:5058–5064, 1995

Ban, E., Crumeyrolle-Arias, M., Latouche, J., *Mol. Cell. Endocrinol* 70:99–107, 1990

Barberis, C., Tribollet, E. Vasopressin and oxytocin receptors in the central nervous system. *Crit. Rev. Neurobiol.* 10:119–154, 1996

Barry, C., Pearson, C., Barbarese, E. Morphological organization of oligodendrocyte processes during development in culture and in vivo. *Dev. Neurosci.* 18:233–242, 1996

Baulieu, E. Contragestion and other clinical applications of RU 486, an antiprogesterone at the receptor. *Science* 245:1351–1356, 1989

Baulieu, E. Neurosteroids of the nervous system, by the nervous system, for the nervous system. *Recent Prog. Horm. Res.* 52:1–32, 1996

Baulieu, E., Schumacher, M., Koenig, H., et al. Progesterone as a neurosteroid: Actions within the nervous system. *Cell. Mol. Neurobiol.* 16:143–154, 1996

Beach, F.A. Importance of progesterone to induction of sexual receptivity in spayed female rats. *Proc. Soc. Exp. Biol. Med.* 51:369–371, 1942

Beach, F.A. *Hormones and Behavior.* New York: Hoeber Harber, 1948

Behl, C., Widmann, M., Trappand, T., Holsboer, F. 17-Beta estradiol protects neurons from oxidative stress-induced cell death in vitro. *Biochem. Biophys. Res. Commun.* 216:473–478, 1996

Bentley, G., Goldsmith A., et al. Photorefractoriness in European starlings (sturnus vulgaris) is not dependent upon the long-day-induced rise in plasma thyroxine. *Gen. Comp. Endocrinol.* 107:428–438, 1997

Bicknell, R.J., Leng, G., Lincoln, D.W., Russell, J.K. Naloxone excites oxytocin neurons in the supraoptic nucleus of lactating rats after chronic morphine treatment. *J. Physiol.* 396:297–317, 1988

Bitran, D., Hilvers, R.J., Kellogg, C.K. Anxiolytic effects of 3a[b]-pregnan-20-one: Endogenous metabolites of progesterone that are active at the GABA$_A$ receptor. *Brain Res.* 561:157–161, 1991

Bitran, D., Purdy, R.H., Kellogg, C.K. Anxiolytic effect of progesterone is associated with increases in cortical allopregnanolone and GABA$_A$ receptor function. *Pharmacol. Biochem. Behav.* 45:423–428, 1993

Bodnar, R., Commons, K., Pfaff, D. Central motive states relating sex and pain. 1999, ms in preparation.

Bolles, R.C. *Theory of motivation.* New York: Harper & Row, 1967

Bolles, R.C. *Theory of motivation (2nd ed.).* New York: Harper & Row, 1975

Bonsall, R.W., Zumpe, D., Michael, R.P. Menstrual cycle influences on operant behavior of female rhesus monkeys. *J. Comp. Physiol. Psychol.* 92:846–855, 1978

Boorstin, D.J. *The Discoverers.* New York: Random House, 1983

Bossmar, T., Forsling, M., Akerlund, M. Circulating oxytocin and vasopressin is influenced by ovarian steroid replacement in women. *Acta Obstet. Gynecol. Scand.* 74:544–548, 1995

Breton, C., Zingg, H.H. Expression and region-specific regulation of the oxytocin receptor gene in rat brain. *Endocrinology* 138:1857–1862, 1997

Brink, E.E., Modianos, D.T., Pfaff, D.W. Ablations of lumbar epaxial musculature: Effects on lordosis behavior of female rats. *Brain Behav. Evol.* 17:67–88, 1980

Brink, E.E., Morrell, J.I., Pfaff, D.W. Localization of lumbar epaxial motoneurons in the rat. *Brain Res.* 170:23–41, 1979

Brink, E.E., Pfaff, D.W. Supraspinal and segmental influence on medial and lateral longissimus nerve activity in rats [abstract 1214]. *Soc. Neurosci. Abstr.* 5:364, 1979

Brink, E.E., Pfaff, D.W. Supraspinal and segmental input to lumbar epaxial motoneurons in the rat. *Brain Res.* 226:43–60, 1981

Brodal, A., Pompeiano, O., Walberg, F. *The vestibular nuclei and their connections, anatomy and functional correlations.* Springfield, IL: Thomas, 1962

Bronson, F.H. *Mammalian reproductive biology.* Chicago: University of Chicago Press, 1989

Brown, H.E., Parhar, I.S., Brooks, P.J., Pfaff, D.W. Estrogen's induction of preproenkephalin (PPE) mRNA in ventromedial hypothalamus (VMN) of female rats is not augmented by voluntary exercise [abstract 202.11]. *Soc. Neurosci. Abstr.* 19:485, 1993

Brown, T.J., Blaustein, J.D. Inhibition of sexual behavior in female guinea pigs by a progestin receptor antagonist. *Brain Res.* 301:343–349, 1984

Buck, L.B. Information coding in the vertebrate olfactory system. *Annu. Rev. Neurosci.* 19:517–544, 1996

Bueno, J., Pfaff, D.W. Single unit recording in hypothalamus and preoptic area of estrogen-treated and untreated ovariectomized female rats. *Brain Res.* 101:67–78, 1976

Burbach, J.P.H., Adan, R.A.H., van Tol, H.H.M., et al. Regulation of the rat oxytocin gene by estradiol. *J. Neuroendocrinol.* 2:633–639, 1990

Butcher, R.L., Collins, W.E., Fugo, N.W. Plasma concentration of LH, FSH, prolactin, progesterone and estradiol-17β throughout the 4-day estrous cycle of the rat. *Endocrinology* 94:1704–1708, 1974

Carlson, H. Observations on stretch reflexes in lumbar back muscles of the cat. *Acta Physiol. Scand.* 103:437–445, 1978

Carrer, H.F., Aoki, A. Ultrastructural changes in the hypothalamic ventromedial nucleus of ovariectomized rats after estrogen treatment. *Brain Res.* 240:221–233, 1982

Carter, C.S., Altemus, M. Integrative functions of lactational hormones in social behavior and stress management. *Ann. N.Y. Acad. Sci.* 807:164–174, 1997

Carter, C.S., DeVries, A.C., Taymans, S.E., et al. Peptides, steroids, and pair bonding. *Ann. N.Y. Acad. Sci.* 807:260–272, 1997a

Carter, C.S., Lederhendler, I.I., Kirkpatrick, B. (Eds.). The integrative neurobiology of affiliation. *Ann. N.Y. Acad. Sci.* 807, 1997b

Carter, C.S., Williams, J., Witt, D., Insel, R. Oxytocin and social bonding. *Ann. N.Y. Acad. Sci.* 652:204–211, 1992

Chalmers, D. *The conscious mind: In search of a fundamental theory.* New York: Oxford University Press, 1996

Chandran, U.R., Attardi, B., Friedman, R., et al. Glucocorticoid repression of the mouse gonadotropin-releasing hormone gene is mediated by promoter elements that are recognized by heteromeric complexes containing glucocorticoid receptor. *J. Biol. Chem.* 271:20412–20420, 1996

Chiapetta, C., Murthy, L., Stancel, G., Hyder, S. The pure antiestrogen ICI 182, 780 differentially inhibits induction of two estrogen regulated genes, *c-fos* and vascular endothelial growth factor [abstract P3-416]. *Endo '97* 540, 1997

———

Chow, S., Sakai, R., Witcher, J., et al. Sex and sodium intake. *Behav. Neurosci.* 106(1):172–180, 1992

Chritin, M., Ueta, Y., Yamashita, K., et al. Vasopressin, oxytocin and angiotensin II receptors in the brain of inbred polydipsic mice [abstract 246.15] *J. Soc. Neurosci.* 22:618, 1996

Chung, S.K., Cohen, R.S., Pfaff, D.W. Ultrastructure and enzyme digestion of nucleoli and associated structures in hypothalamic nerve cells viewed in resinless sections. *Biol. Cell.* 51:23–34, 1984

Chung, S.K., Haldar, J., Pfaff, D.W. *Estrogen effect on oxytocin mRNA-expressing neurons which project to spinal cord studied by combination of in situ hybridization and retrograde marker. Manuscript* submitted for publication

Chung, S.K., McCabe, J.T., Pfaff, D.W. Estrogen influences on oxytocin mRNA expression in preoptic and anterior hypothalamic regions studied by in situ hybridization. *J. Comp. Neurol.* 307:281–395, 1991

Chung, S.K., Pfaff, D.W., Cohen, R.S. Estrogen-induced alterations in synaptic morphology in the midbrain central gray. *Exp. Brain Res.* 69:522–530, 1988

Chung, S.K., Pfaff, D.W., Cohen, R.S. Projections of ventromedial hypothalamic neurons to the midbrain central gray: An ultrastructural study. *Neuroscience* 38:395–407, 1990a

Chung, S.K., Pfaff, D.W., Cohen, R.S. Transneuronal degeneration in the midbrain central gray following chemical lesions in the ventromedial nucleus: A qualitative and quantitative analysis. *Neuroscience* 38:409–426, 1990b

Cohen, M.S., Schwartz-Giblin, S., Pfaff, D.W. Brainstem reticular stimulation facilitates back muscle motoneuronal responses to pudendal nerve input. *Brain Res.* 405:155–158, 1987b

Cohen, R.S., Chung, S.R., Pfaff, D.W. Alteration by estrogen of the nucleoli in nerve cells of the rat hypothalamus. *Cell Tissue Res.* 235:485–489, 1984

Cohen, R.S., Chung, S.R., Pfaff, D.W. Immunocytochemical localization of actin in dendritic spines of the cerebral cortex using colloidal gold as a probe. *Cell. Mol. Neurobiol.* 5(3): 271–284, 1985a

Cohen, R.S., Pfaff, D.W. Ultrastructure of neurons in the ventromedial nucleus of the hypothalamus in ovariectomized rats with or without estrogen treatment. *Cell Tissue Res.* 217: 451–470, 1981

Cohen, R.S., Pfaff, D.W. Cell biological and math-logical theories of the neural circuit for steroid-dependent female reproductive behavior. *Integ. Psychiatry* 3:262–279, 1985b

Cohen, R.S., Pfaff, D.W. Cytology and organization of cell types: Light and electron microscopy. In P.M. Conn (Ed.), *Neuroscience in medicine.* Philadelphia: Lippincott, 1995: 21–36

Cohen, R.S., Pfaff, D.W. Ventromedial hypothalamic neurons in the mediation of long-lasting effects of estrogen on lordosis behavior. *Prog. Neurobiol.* 38:423–453, 1992

Conrad, L.C.A., Pfaff, D.W. Efferents from medial basal forebrain and hypothalamus in the rat: I. An autoradiography study of the medial preoptic area. *J. Comp. Neurol.* 169:185–220, 1976a

Conrad, L.C.A., Pfaff, D.W. Efferents from medial basal forebrain and hypothalamus in the rat: II. An autoradiography study of the anterior hypothalamus. *J. Comp. Neurol.* 169:221–262, 1976b

Coirini, H., Johnson, A.E., McEwen, B.S. Estradiol modulation of oxytocin binding in the ventromedial hypothalamic nucleus of male and female rats. *Neuroendocrinology* 50:193–198, 1989

Cottingham, S.L., Femano, P.A., Pfaff, D.W. Electrical stimulation of the midbrain central gray facilitates reticulospinal activation of axial muscle EMG. *Exp. Neurol.* 97:704–724, 1987

Cottingham, S.L., Femano, P.A., Pfaff, D.W. Vestibulospinal and reticulospinal interactions in the activation of back muscle EMG in the rat. *Exp. Brain Res.* 73:198–208, 1988

Cottingham, S.L., Pfaff, D.W. Interconnectedness of steroid hormone–binding neurons: Existence and implications. *Curr. Top. Neuroendocrinol.* 7:223–250, 1986

Cottingham, S.L., Pfaff, D.W. Electrical stimulation of the midbrain central gray facilitates lateral vestibulospinal activation of back muscle EMG in the rat. *Brain Res.* 421:397–400, 1987

Crick, F.H.C. The genetic code. *Sci. Am.* 66–74, 1962

Crowley, W.R., Kalra, S.P. Neuropeptide Y stimulates the release of luteinizing hormone-releasing hormone from medial basal hypothalamus in vitro: Modulation by ovarian hormones. *Neuroendocrinology* 46:97–103, 1987

Dahl, G., Evans N., et al. Thyroxine is permissive to seasonal transitions in reproductive neuroendocrine activity in the ewe. *Biol. Reprod.* 52:690–696, 1995

Dahlström, A., Fuxe, K. Evidence for the existence of monoamine containing neurons in the central nervous system: I. Demonstration of monoamines in the cell bodies of brainstem neurons. *Acta. Physiol. Scand.* 62 (Suppl. 232): 1–55, 1964

Daly, E., Gray, A., Barlow, D., et al. Measuring the impact of menopausal symptoms on quality of life. *Br. Med. J.* 307:836–840, 1993

Daniel, J., Dohanich, G. Effects of varying periods of estrogen exposure on the acquisition of a radial arm maze by female rats. *Soc. Behav. Neuroendocrinol.* p. 132, 1997

Davis, G.A., Moore, F.L. Neuroanatomical distribution of androgen and estrogen receptor–immunoreactive cells in the brain of the male roughskin newt. *J. Com. Neurol.* 372:294–308, 1996

Davis, P.G., Krieger, M.S., Barfield, R.J., et al. The site of action of intrahypothalamic estrogen implants in feminine sexual behavior: An autoradiography analysis. *Endocrinology* 111: 1581–1586, 1982

Davis, S.R., Burger, H.G. Androgens and the postmenopausal woman. *J. Clin. Endocrinol. Metab.* 81:2759–2763, 1996

de Jonge, F.H., Burger, J., van Haaren, F., et al. Sexual experience and preference for males or females in the female rat. *Behav. Neural Biol.* 47:369–383, 1987

Dellovade, T.L., Hardelin, J., Soussi-Yanicostas, N., et al. *Ansomin-I immunoreactivity during embryogenesis in a primitive eutherian mammal.* Manuscript submitted for publication

Dellovade, T.L., Zhu, Y.-S., Krey, L., Pfaff, D.W. Thyroid hormone and estrogen interact to regulate behavior. *Proc. Natl. Acad. Sci.* 93:12581–12586, 1996

Dellovade, T.L., Zhu, Y.-S., Pfaff, D.W. Potential interactions between estrogen receptor and thyroid receptor relevant for neuroendocrine systems. *J. Steroid Biochem. Mol. Biol.* 53:27–31, 1995a

Dellovade, T.L., Zhu, Y.-S., Pfaff, D.W. Thyroid hormone and estradiol alter oxytocin gene expression in the paraventricular nucleus [abstract 80.5]. *J. Soc. Neurosci.* 21:189, 1995b

Dellovade, T.L., Zhu, Y.S., Pfaff, D.W. Thyroid hormone and estrogen affect oxytocin gene expression in hypothalamic neurons. *J. Neuroendocrinol.,* 1999 in press

Delville, W., Mansour, K.M., Ferris, C.F. Testosterone facilitates aggression by modulating vasopressin receptors in the hypothalamus. *Physiol. Behav.* 60:25–29, 1996

Dluzen, D.E., McDermottand, J.L., Liu, B. Estrogen as a neuroprotectant against MPTP-induced neurotoxicity in C57/B1 mice. *Neurotoxicicol. Teratol.* 18:603–606, 1996

Dohanich, G., Fader, A., Daniel, J., et al. Estrogen regulation of learning and memory. *Soc. Behav. Neuroendocrinol.* 47, 1997

Dollard, J.C., Miller, N.E. *Personality and psychotherapy.* New York: McGraw-Hill, 1950

Douglas, A.J., Antonijevic, I.A., Neumann, I., Russell, J.A. The key role of maternal neurohypophysial oxytocin in parturition. In K. Maeda, H. Tsukamura, A. Yokoyama, (Eds.), *Neural control of reproduction: Physiology and behavior.* Tokyo: Japan Scientific Societies Press, 1997:121–133

Douglas, A.J., Bicknell, R.J. Russell, J.A. Pathways to parturition. In R. Ivell, J.A. Russell *Oxytocin: Cellular and molecular approaches in medicine and research,* Vol. 395. New York: Plenum, 1995b:381–394

Douglas, A.J., Dye, S., Leng, G., et al. Endogenous opioid regulation of oxytocin secretion through pregnancy in the rat. *J. Neuroendocrinol.* 5:307–314, 1993

Douglas, A.J., Neumann, I., Meeren, H.K.M., et al. Central endogenous opioid inhibition of supraoptic oxytocin neurons in pregnant rats. *J. Neurosci.* 15:5049–5057, 1995a

Dudley, C.A., Vale, W., Rivier,J., Moss, R.L. The effect of LHRH antagonist analogs and an antibody to LHRH on mating behavior in female rats. *Peptides* 2:393–396, 1981

Dudley, C.A., Vale, W., Rivier, J., Moss, R.L. Facilitation of sexual receptivity in the female rat by a fragment of the LHRH decapeptide, Ac-LHRH. *Neuroendocrinology* 36:486–488, 1983

Dulac, C., Axel, R. A novel family of genes encoding putative pheromone receptors in mammals. *Cell* 83:195–206, 1995

Endicott, J., Halbreich, U. Retrospective report of premenstrual depressive changes: Factors affecting confirmation by daily ratings. *Psychopharmacol. Bull.* 18(3):109–112, 1982

Etgen, A. Antiestrogens: Effects of tamoxifen, nafoxidine and CI-628 on sexual behavior, cytoplasmic receptors and nuclear binding of receptors. *Horm. Behav.* 13:97—112, 1979

Etgen, A., Barfield R. Antagonism of female sexual behavior with intracerebral implants of antiprogestin RU 38486: Corresatin with binding to neural progestin receptors. *Endocrinology* 119:1610–1617, 1986

Everts, H., De Ruiter, A., Koolhass, J. Differential lateral septal vasopressin in wild-type rats: Correlation with aggression. *Horm. Behav.* 31:136–144, 1997

Fader, A., Wolff, S., Dohanich, G. Estrogen reversal of amnestic effects of scopolamine administered to the hippocampus. *Soc. Behav. Neuroendocrinol.* 133, 1997

Fahrbach, S.E., Morrell, J.I., Pfaff, D.W. Effect of varying the duration of pre-test cage habituation on oxytocin induction of short-latency maternal behavior. *Physiol. Behav.* 37:135–139, 1986

Fernandez-Gausti, A., Picazo, O. Changes in burying behavior during the estrous cycle: Effect of estrogen and progesterone. *Psychoneuroendocrinology* 17:681–689, 1992

Ferris C.F. Role of vasopressin in aggressive and dominant/subordinate behaviors. *Ann. N.Y. Acad. Sci.* 652:212–226, 1992

Ferris, C.F., Delville, Y. Vasopressin and serotonin interactions in the control of agonistic behavior. *Psychoneuroendocrinology* 19:593–601, 1994

Ferris, C.F., Pan, J.X., Singer, E.A., et al. Stimulation of luteinizing hormone release after steriotaxic microinjection of neurotensin into the medial preoptic area of rats. *Neuroendocrinology* 38:144–151, 1984

Ferster, C.B., Skinner, B.F. *Schedules of reinforcement.* New York: Appleton-Century-Crofts; 1957

Fink, G. Hypothalamic pituitary ovarian axis. In J. Stallworthy, G. Bourne (Eds.), *Recent advances in obstetrics and gynaecology,* Vol. 12. Edinburgh: Churchill Livingstone, 1977

Fink, G. The psychoprotective action of estrogen is mediated by central serotonergic as well as dopaminergic mechanisms. In A. Takada, G. Curzon (Eds.), *Serotonin in the central nervous system and periphery.* Amsterdam: Elsevier Science, 1995

Fink, G., Sumner, B., Rosie, R., et al. Estrogen control of central neurotransmission: Effect on mood, mental state, and memory. *Cell. Mol. Neurobiol.* 16:325–344,1996

Fisher, H.E. Lust, attraction and attachment in mammalian reproduction. *Hum. Nature* (in press)

Floody, O.R., Pfaff, D.W. Communication among hamsters by high-frequency acoustic signals: III. Responses evoked by natural and synthetic ultrasounds. *J. Comp. Physiol. Psychol.* 91:820–829, 1977

———

Flugge, G., Oertel, W.H., Wuttke, W. Evidence for estrogen-receptive GABAergic neurons in the preoptic/anterior hypothalamic area of the rat brain. *Neuroendocrinology* 43:1–5, 1986

Fluharty, S., Sakai, R. Behavioral and cellular analysis of adrenal steroid and angiotensin interactions mediating salt appetite. *Prog. Psychobiol. Physiol. Psychology* 16:177–212, 1995

Franco, B., Balabio, A., et al. A gene deleted in Kallmann's syndrome shares homology with neural cell adhesion and axonal path-finding molecules. *Nature* 353:529–536, 1991

Frankfurt, M., Gonadal steroids and neuronal plasticity: Studies in the adult rat hypothalamus. *Ann. N.Y. Acad. Sci.* 743:45–60, 1994

Frankfurt, M., Gould, E., Wooley, C.S., McEwen, B.S. Gonadal steroids modify dendritic spine density in ventromedial hypothalamic neurons: A golgi study in the adult rat. *Neuroendocrinology* 51:531–535, 1990

Frankfurt, M., McEwen, B.S. 5,7-Dihydroxytryptamine and gonadal steroid manipulation alter spine density in ventromedial hypothalamic neurons. *Neuroendocrinology* 54:653–657, 1991

Freeman, E.W., Purdy, R.H., Coutifaris, C., et al. Anxiolytic metabolites of progesterone: Correlation with mood and performance measures following oral progesterone administration to healthy female volunteers. *Neuroendocrinology* 58:478–484, 1993

Freud, S., *Instincts and their vicissitudes,* Vol. 14. 117–140

Freud, S. *Three essays on the theory of sexuality,* Vol. 7. New York: Basic Books, 1962:125–245 (orig. pub. 1905)

Funabashi, T., Brooks, P.J., Kleopoulus, S.P., et al. Changes in preproenkephalin messenger RNA level in the rat ventromedial hypothalamus during the estrous cycle. *Mol. Brain Res.* 28:129–134, 1995

Funabashi, T., Brooks, P.J., Mobbs, C.V., Pfaff, D.W. DNA methylation and DNase-hypersensitive sites in the 5′ flanking and transcribed regions of the rat preproenkephalin gene: Studies of mediobasal hypothalamus. *Mol. Cell. Neurosci.* 4:499–509, 1993

Funabashi, T., Brooks, P.J., Weesner G.D., Pfaff D.W. Luteinizing hormone-releasing hormone receptor messenger ribonucleic acid expression in the rat pituitary during lactation and the estrous cycle. *J. Neuroendocrinol.* 6:261–266, 1994

Fuxe, K. Evidence for the existence of monoamine containing neurons in the central nervous system: IV. The distribution of monoamine terminals in the central nervous system. *Acta Physiol. Scand. Suppl.* 64:247, 1965

Fuxe, K., Gunne, L.M. *Acta Physiol. Scand. Suppl.* 62:493, 1964

Fuxe, K., Hamberger, B., Hokfelt, T. Distribution of noradrenaline nerve terminals in cortical areas of the rat. *Brain Res.* 8:125–131, 1968

Fuxe, K., Hökfelt, T. *Acta Physiol. Scand.* 66:245, 1966

Fuxe, K., Hökfelt, T. In W.F. Ganong, L. Martini (Eds.), *Frontiers in neuroendocrinology.* New York: Oxford University Press, 1969:47

Fuxe, K., Hökfelt, T., Ungerstedt, U. Morphological and functional aspects of central monoamine neurons. *Int. Rev. Neurobiol.* 13:93–126, 1970

Garcia-Estrada, J., Del Rio, J.A., Luquin, S., et al. Gonadal hormones down-regulate reactive gliosis and astrocyte proliferation after a penetrating brain injury. *Brain Res.* 628:271–278, 1993

Gardner, H. *Frames of mind: The theory of multiple intelligence.* New York: Basic Books, 1983

Geissler, W.M., Davis, D.L., Wu, L., et al. Male pseudohermaphroditism caused by mutations of testicular 17β-hydroxysteroid dehydrogenase 3. *Nature Genet* 7:34–39, 1994

Gerlach, J., McEwen, B., Pfaff, D., et al. Cells in regions of rhesus monkey brain and pituitary retain radioactive estradiol, corticosterone and cortisol differentially. *Brain Res.* 103:603–612, 1976

Getchell, M. L., Kulkarni-Narla, R., Marcinek, R., Getchell, T.V. Estrogen receptors are expressed in olfactory and vomeronasal receptor neurons. *J. Soc. Neurosci.* 22:1594, 1996

Gibbs, R., Burke, A., Johnson, D. Effects of estrogen replacement on lorazepam- and scopolamine-induced impairments in passive avoidance memory. *Soc. Behav. Neuroendocrinol.* 134, 1997

Gibson, M.J., Moscovitz, H.C., Kokoris, G.J., Silverman, A.J. Female sexual behavior in hypogonadal mice with GnRH containing brain grafts. *Horm. Behav.* 21:211–222, 1987

Glaser, J., Barfield, R. Blockade of progesterone-activated estrous behavior in rats by intracerebral anisomycin is site specific. *Neuroendocrinology* 38:337–343, 1984

Goldsmith, A. and Nichols, T. Thyroidectomy prevents the development of photorefractoriness and the associated rise in plasma prolactin in starlings. *Gen. Comp. Endocrinol.* 54: 256–263, 1984a

Goldsmith, A. and Nichols, T. Thyroxine induces photorefractoriness and stimulates prolactin secretion in European starlings (sturnus vulgaris). *J. Endocrinol.* 101:1–3, 1984b

Goleman, D. *Emotional intelligence.* New York: Bantam Books, 1995

Goodman, Y., Bruce, A.J., Chengand, B., Mattson, M.P. Estrogens attenuate and corticosterone exacerbates excitotoxicity, oxidative injury, and amyloid beta-peptide toxicity in hippocampal neurons. *J. Neurochem.* 66:1836–1844, 1996

Gordan, J., Attardi, B., Pfaff, D.W. Mathematical exploration of pulsatility in GT-1 cells. *Neuroendocrinology* (in press)

Gould, J.L. *Ethology: The mechanisms and evolution of behavior.* New York: Norton, 1982

Gould, E., Woolley, C.S., Frankfurt, M., McEwen, B.S. Gonadal steroids regulate dendritic spine density in hippocampal pyramidal cells in adulthood. *Neurosci.* 10:1286–1291, 1990

Goy, R., McEwen, B. *Sexual differentiation of the brain*. Cambridge, MA: MIT Press, 1980

Green, P.S., Gridley, K.E., Simpkins, J.W. Estradiol protects against beta-amyloid (25-35)-induced toxicity in SK-N-SH human neuroblastoma cells. *Neurosci. Let.* 218:165–168, 1996

Gregory, E., Engel, K., Pfaff, P. Male hamster preference for odors of female hamster vaginal discharges: Studies of experiental and hormonal determinants. *Comp. Physiol. Psychology* 89:442–446, 1975

Grillner, S., Hongo, T., Lund, S. The vestibulospinal tract. Effects on alpha-motoneurones in the lumbosacral spinal cord in the cat. *Exp. Brain Res.* 10:94–120, 1970

Grillner, S., Hongo, T., Lund, S. Convergent effects on alpha motoneurones from the vestibulospinal tract and a pathway descending I the medial longitudinal fasciculus. *Exp. Brain Res.* 12:457–479, 1971

Gross, P., Ritcher, D., Robertson, G.L. *Vasopressin*. Paris: John Libby Eurotext, 1993

Halbreich, U., Endicott, J., Goldstein, S., Nee, J. Premenstrual changes and changes in gonadal hormones. *Acta Psychiatr. Scand.* 74:576–586, 1986

Halbreich, U., Endicott, J., Lesser, J. The clinical diagnosis and classification of premenstrual changes. *Can. J. Psychiatry* 30:489–97, 1985

Haqq, C., Donahoe, P. Regulation of sexual dimorphism in mammals. *Physiol. Rev.* 78(1): 1–33, 1998

Hardy, R., Friedrich, V. Progressive remodeling of the oligodendrocyte process arbor during myelinogenesis. *Dev. Neurosci.* 18:243–254, 1996

Harlan, R.E., Shivers, B.D., Romano, G.J., et al. Location of preproenkephalin mRNA in the rat brain and spinal cord by in situ hybridization. *J. Comp. Neurol.* 258:159–184, 1987

Hasegawa, T., Sakuma, Y. *Brain Res.* 611:1–6, 1993

Hassen, A., Barnes, C. Bilateral effects of vestibular nerve stimulation on activity in the lumbar spinal cord. *Brain Res.* 90:221–233, 1975

Heierhorst, J., Lederis, K., Richter, D. Vasotocin neuropeptide precursors and genes of teleost and jawless fish. In Hochachka, H., & Mommsen J. (Eds.), *Biochemistry and molecular biology of fishes, Vol. 2*. Amsterdam: Elsevier, 1993:339–355

Heierhorst, J., Morely, S., Figueroa, J., Krentler, C., Lederis, K., Richter, D. Vasotocin and isotocin precursors from the white sucker, *Catostomus commersoni:* Cloning and sequence analysis of the cDNAs. *Proc. Natl. Acad. Sci. U.S.A.* 86:5242–5246, 1989

Henderson, V.W., Paganini-Hill, A., Emanuel, C.K., et al. Estrogen replacement therapy in older women: Comparisons between Alzheimer's disease cases and nondemented control subjects. *Arch. Neurol.* 51:896–900, 1994

Herbison, A.E. Estrogen regulation of cyclic GnRH secretion. *Rev. Reprod.* 1:1–6, 1997

Herbison, A.E., Simonian, S.X. Characterization of brainstem of estrogen-receptive neurons projecting to the vicinity of the gonadotrophin-releasing hormone (GnRH) cell bodies in the rat [abstract 624.16]. *Soc. Neurosci. Abstr.* 22:1996

Herrnstein, R., Murray, C. *The bell curve*. New York: Free Press, 1994

Hinde, R. *Animal behavior: A synthesis of ethology and comparative psychology* (2nd ed.). New York: McGraw-Hill, 1966.

Hökfelt, T. *Experientia* 22:56, 1966

Hökfelt, T. On the ultrastructural localization of noradrenaline in the central nervous system of the rat. *Z. Zellforsch. Mikroskop. Anat.* 79:110, 1967a

Hökfelt, T. The possible ultrastructural identification of tubero-infundibular dopamine-containing nerve endings in the median eminence of the rat. *Brain Res.* 5:121, 1967b

Hökfelt, T. In vitro studies on central and peripheral monoamine neurons at the ultrastructural level. *Z. Zellforsch. Mikroskop. Anat.* 91:1, 1968a.

Hökfelt, T. *Unpublished doctoral thesis, Karolinska Institutet, Stockholm* 1968b

Hökfelt, T. Distribution of noradrenaline storing particles in peripheral adrenergic neurons as revealed by electron microscopy. *Acta Physiol. Scand.* 76:427, 1969

Hökfelt, T., Fuxe, K. *Exp. Brain Res.* 9:63, 1969a

Hökfelt, T., Ljungdahl, Å., Fuxe, K., Johansson, O. Dopamine nerve terminals in the rat limbic cortex: Aspects of the dopamine hypothesis of schizophrenia. *Science* 184:177–179, 1974

Hökfelt, T., Ungersatedt, U. *Acta Physiol. Scand.* 76:415, 1969b

Holtzman, D.A., Brooks, P.J., Pfaff, D.W., Schwartz-Giblin, S. Preproenkephalin mRNA expression in the ventromedial nucleus of the hypothalamus and lumbar dorsal horn of female rats following gonadal steroids and formalin injection [abstract 576.6]. *Soc. Neurosci. Abstr.* 18:1372, 1992

Holtzman, D.A., Brooks, P.J., Pfaff, D.W., Schwartz-Giblin, S. Preproenkephalin mRNA expression is regulated by an interaction between steroid hormones and nociceptive stimulation. *J. Neuroendocrinology* 9:913–922, 1997

Holzbauer, M. In vivo production of steroids with central depressant actions by the ovary of the rat. *Br. J. Pharmacol.* 43:560–569, 1971

Hongo, T., Kudo, N., Tanaka, R. The vestibulospinal tract: Crossed and uncrossed effects on hindlimb motoneurones in the cat. *Exp. Brain Res.* 24:37–55, 1975

Honjo, H., Tamura, T., Matsumoto, Y., et al. Estrogen as a growth factor to central nervous cells. Estrogen treatment promotes development of acetylcholinesterase-positive basal forebrain neurons transplanted in the anterior eye chamber. *J. Steroid Biochem Mol. Biol.* 41: 633–635, 1992

Horton, R. Testicular steroid secretions, metabolism, and mode of action. In L.J. DeGroot (Ed.), *Endocrinology,* Vol. 3. Philadelphia: Saunders, 1989:2146–2151

Hull, C.L., *Principles of behavior.* New York: Appleton-Century-Crofts, 1943

Hyder, S.M., Stancel, G.M., Chiappetta, C., et al. Uterine expression of vascular endothelial growth factor is increased by estradiol tamoxifen. *Cancer Res.* 56:3954–3960, 1996

Imperato-McGinley J., Peterson, R.E., Gautier, T., Sturla, E. Androgens and the evolution of male-gender identity among male pseudohermaphrodites with 5α-reductase deficiency. *N. Engl. J. Med.* 300:1233–1237, 1979

Imura, H. Endocrine and metabolic manifestations associated with infectious and inflammatory diseases. *FEMS Immuno. Med. Microbio.* 18(4):221–226, 1997

Insel, T.R., Shapiro, L.E. Oxytocin receptors and maternal behavior. *Ann. N.Y. Acad. Sci.* 652:122–141, 1992a

Insel, T.R., Shapiro, L.E. Oxytocin receptor distribution reflects social organization in monogamous and polygamous voles. *Proc. Natl. Acad. Sci. U.S.A.* 89:5981–5985, 1992b

Ivell, R., Richter, D. Structure and comparison of the oxytocin and vasopressin genes from rat. *Proc. Natl. Acad. Sci. U.S.A.* 81:2006–2010, 1984

Jennes, L., Brame, B., Centers, A., et al. *Mol. Brain Res.* 33:104–110, 1995

Jennes, L., Centers, A. Changes in gonadotropin releasing hormone receptor (GnRH-R) mRNA content of the rat mediobasal hypothalamus during the estrogen-progesterone induced JH surge [abstract 379.11]. *J. Soc. Neurosci.* 22:959, 1996

Jennes, L., McShane, T.M., Brame, B., Centers, A. *J. Neuroendocrinol.* 8:275–281, 1996a

Jennes, L., Ozhan, E., Janovick, J.A., Conn, P.M. Brain gonadotropin releasing hormone receptors: Localization and regulation. *Recent Prog. Horm. Res.* 52:475–491, 1996b

Jiang, N., Chopp, M. Progesterone is neuroprotective after transient middle cerebral artery occlusion in male rats. *Brain Res.* 735:101, 1996

Jirikowski, G.F., Caldwell, J.D., Stumpf, W.E., Pedersen, C.A. Estradiol influences oxytocin immunoreactive brain systems. *Neuroscience* 25:237–248, 1988

Johnson, A.E., Coirini, H., McEwen, B.S., Insel, T.R. Testosterone modulates oxytocin binding in the hypothalamus of castrated male rats. *Neuroendocrinology* 50:199–203, 1989

Jones, K.J., Chikaraishi, D.M., Harrington, C.A., et al. In situ hybridization detection of estradiol-induced changes in ribosomal RNA levels in rat brain. *Mol. Brain Res.* 1:145–152, 1986a

Jones, K.J., Harrington, C.A., Chikaraishi, D.M., Pfaff, D.W. Steroid hormone regulation of ribosomal RNA in rat hypothalamus: Early detection using *in situ* hybridization and precursor-product ribosomal DNA probes. *J. Neurosci.* 10(5):1513–1521, 1990

Jones, K.J., McEwen, B.S., Pfaff, D.W. Quantitative assessment of the synergistic and independent effects of estradiol and progesterone on ventromedial hypothalamic and preoptic-area proteins in female rat brain. *Metab. Brain Dis.* 2:271–281, 1987

Jones, K.J., McEwen, B.S., Pfaff, D.W. Quantitative assessment of early and discontinuous estradiol-induced effects on ventromedial hypothalamic and preoptic area proteins in female rat brain. *Neuroendocrinology* 48:561–568, 1988

Jones, K.J., McEwen, B.S., Pfaff, D.W. Regional specificity in estradiol effects on [3H]uridine incorporation in rat brain. *Mol. Cell. Endocrinol.* 45:57–63, 1986b

Jones, K.J., Pfaff, D.W. Emerging tenets in the mechanism of gonadal steroid action on hypothalamic neurons. In M. Motta (Ed.), *Brain Endocrinology (2nd ed.)*. New York: Raven Press, 1991

Jones, K.J., Pfaff, D.W., McEwen, B.S. Early estrogen-induced nuclear changes in rat hypothalamic ventromedial neurons: An ultrastructural and morphometric analysis. *J. Comp. Neurol.* 239:255–266, 1985

Jones, K.J., Pfaff, D.W., McEwen, B.S. Ultrastructural and morphometric analysis of neurons in the arcuate nucleus of the female rat hypothalamus following estradiol. *Brain Res. Bull.* 26:181–184, 1991

Jonkalass, J., Buggy, J. Angiotensin-estrogen interaction in female brain reduces drinking and pressor responses. *Am. J. Physiol.* 247:R167–R172, 1984

Jonkalass, J., Buggy, J. Angiotensin-estrogen central interactions: Localization and mechanisms. *Brain Res.* 326:239–249, 1985

Jung-Testas, I., Hu, Z.Y., Baulieu, E., Robel, P. *Endocrinology.* 125:2083–2091, 1989

Jung-Testas, I., Renoir, J., Gasc, J., Baulieu, E. *Exp. Cell Res.* 193:12–19, 1991

Kampen, D.L., Sherwin, B.B. Estrogen use and verbal memory in healthy postmenopausal women. *Obstet. Gynecol.* 83:979–983, 1994

Kampen, D.L., Sherwin, B.B. Estradiol is related to visual memory in healthy young men. *Behav. Neurosci.* 110:613–617, 1996

Kandel, E.R. *The behavioral biology of aplysia: A contribution to the comparative study of opisthobranch molluscs.* San Francisco: Freeman, 1979

Kandel, E.R., Schwartz, J.H. (Eds.). *Principles of neural science* (2nd ed.). New York: Elsevier/North-Holland, 1991

Kaplitt, M.G., Kwong, A.D., Kleopoulos, S.P., et al. Preproenkephalin promoter yields region-specific and longterm expression in adult brain following direct in vivo gene transfer via a defective herpes simplex viral vector. *Proc. Nat'l. Acad. Sci. U.S.A.* 91:8979–8983, 1994

Kaplitt, M.G., Pfaus, J.G., Kleopoulos, S.P., et al. Expression of a functional foreign gene in adult mammalian brain following in vivo transfer via a herpes simplex virus type 1 defective viral vector. *Mol. Cell. Neurosci.* 2:320–330, 1991

Kaplitt, M.G., Rabkin, S., Pfaff, D.W. Molecular alterations in nerve cells: Direct manipulation and physiology mediation. *Curr. Top. Neuroendocrinol.* 2:169–191, 1993

Kawas, C., et al. A prospective study of estrogen replacement therapy and the risk of developing Alzheimer's disease. *Neurology* 48:1517–1521, 1997

Kelley, D.B., Pfaff, D.W. Generalizations from comparative studies on neuroanatomical and endocrine mechanisms of sexual behaviour. In J. Hutchison (Ed.), *Biological determinants of sexual behavior.* Chichester, England: Wiley, 1978:225–254

Keye, W.R., Yuen, B.H., Jaffe, R.B., New concepts in the physiology of the menstrual cycle. *Clin. Endocrinol. Metab.* 2:451–467, 1973

Kimura, D. Estrogen replacement therapy may protect against intellectual decline in postmenopausal women. *Horm. Behav.* 29:312–321, 1995

Kimura, T., Tanizawa, O., Mori, K., et al. *Nature* 356:526–529, 1992

Kindler, S., Mohr, E., Richter, D. Quo vadis: Extrasomatic targeting of neuronal mRNAs in mammals. *Mol. Cell. Endocrinol.* 128(1–2):7–10, 1997

King, J., Anthony, E. LHRH neurons and their projections in humans and other mammals: Species comparisons. *Peptides* 5:195–207, 1984

King, J., Anthony, E., Fitzgerald, D., Stopa, E. Luteinizing hormone-releasing hormone neurons in human preoptic/hypothalamus: Differential intraneuronal localization of immunoreactive forms. *J. Clin. Endocrinol. Metab.* 60:88–97, 1985

Kisley, L., Sakai, R., Ma, L., Fluharty, S. Ovarian steroid regulation of angiotensin II–induced water intake in the rat. *Am. J. Physiol.* in press 1998,

Knobil, E., Neill, J. (Eds.). *The physiology of reproduction* (2nd ed.). New York: Raven Press, 1994

Koenig, H., Schumacher, M., Ferzaz, B., et al. Progesterone synthesis and myelin formation by Schwann cells. *Science* 268:1500–1503, 1995

Kow, L.-M., Brown, H.E., Pfaff, D.W. Activation of protein kinase C in the hypothalamic ventromedial nucleus of the midbrain central gray facilitates lordosis. *Brain Res.* 660:241–248, 1994a

Kow, L.-M., Johnson, A.E., Ogawa, S., Pfaff, D.W. Electrophysiological actions of oxytocin on hypothalamic neurons, in vitro: Neuropharmacological characterization and effects of ovarian steroids. *Neuroendocrinology* 54:526–535, 1991

Kow, L.-M., McEwen, B.S., Pfaff, D.W., Weiland, N.G. G-protein activation in hypothalamic ventromedial nucleus (VMN) by phenylephrine (PhE), and its potentiation by estrogen: Autoradiographic evidence. *Soc. Neurosci. Abstr.* 1997

Kow, L.-M., Mobbs, C.V., Pfaff, D.W. Roles of second-messenger systems and neuronal activity in the regulation of lordosis by neurotransmitters, neuropeptides and estrogen: A review. *Neurosci. Biobehav. Rev.* 18:251–268, 1994b

Kow, L.-M., Montgomery, M.O., Pfaff, D.W. Triggering of lordosis reflex in female rats with somatosensory stimulation: Quantitative determination of stimulus parameters. *J. Neurophysiol.* 42:195–202, 1979

Kow, L.-M., Pfaff, D.W. Effects of estrogen treatment on the size of receptive field and response threshold of pudendal nerve in the female rat. *Neuroendocrinology* 13:299–313, 1973

Kow, L., Pfaff, D. Mapping of neural and signal transduction and pathways for lordosis in the search for estrogen actions on the central nervous system. *Behav. Brain Res.* 92:169–180, 1998

Kow, L.-M., Pfaff, D.W. Responses to single units in sixth lumbar dorsal root ganglion of female rats to mechanostimulation relevant for lordosis reflex. *J. Neurophysiol.* 42:203–213, 1979

Kow, L.-M., Pfaff, D.W. Responses of ventromedial hypothalamic neurons in vitro to norepinephrine; dependence on dose and receptor type. *Brain Res.* 413:220–228, 1987

Kow, L.-M., Pfaff, D.W. Transmitter and peptide actions on hypothalamic neurons in vitro: Implications for lordosis. *Brain Res. Bull.* 20:857–861, 1988

Kow, L.-M., Pfaff, D.W., Ogawa, S. Functional differences between two G protein isoforms, $G\alpha_{11}$ and $G\alpha_q$: Evidence from the use of antisense oligodeoxynucleotides (ODN_S) in the study of lordosis. *Soc. Neurosc. Abstr.* 360.17, p. 919, 1996

Kow, L.-M., Weesner, G.D., Pfaff, D.W. a,-adrenergic agonists act on ventromedial hypothalamic a,b-receptors to cause neuronal excitation and lordosis facilitation: Electrophysiological and behavioral evidence. *Brain Res.* 588:237–245, 1992

Kow, L.-M., Zemlan, F.P., Pfaff, D.W. Responses of lumbosacral spinal units to mechanical stimuli related to analysts of lordosis reflex in female rats. *J. Neurophysiol.* 43:27–45, 1980

Krebs, C.J., Jarvis, E.D., Pfaff, D.W. Characterization of progesterone-responsive genes from the female rat hypothalamus isolated by the differential display polymerase chain reaction. *Soc. Neurosci. Abstr.* 1997.

Krieger, M.S., Conrad, L.C.A., Pfaff, D.W. An autoradiography study of the efferent connections of the ventromedial nucleus of the hypothalamus. *J. Comp. Neurol.* 183:785–816, 1979

Krsmanovic, L.Z., Stojilkovic, S.S., Mertz, L.M., et al. Expression of gonadotropin-releasing hormone receptors and autocrine regulation of neuropeptide release in immortalized hypothalamic neurons. *Proc. Natl. Acad. Sci. U.S.A.* 90:3908–39112, 1993

Kuiper, G.G., Enmark, E., Pelto-Huikko, M., et al. Cloning of a novel receptor expressed in rat prostate and ovary. *Proc. Natl. Acad. Sci. U.S.A.* 93:5925–5930, 1996

Land, H., Schutz, G., Schmale, H., Richter, D. Nucleotide sequence of cloned cDNA encoding the bovine arginine vasopressin/neurophysin II precursor. *Nature* 295:299–303, 1982

Lauber, A.H., Mobbs, C.V., Muramatsu, M., Pfaff, D.W. Estrogen receptor mRNA expression in rat hypothalamus as a function of genetic sex and estrogen dose. *Endocrinology* 129(6):3180–3186, 1991a

Lauber, A.H., Romano, G.J., Mobbs, C.V., et al. Estradiol induction of proenkephalin messenger RNA in hypothalamus: Dose-response and relation to reproductive behavior in the female rat. *Mol. Brain Res.* 8:47–54, 1990a

Lauber, A.H., Romano, G.J., Mobbs, C.V., Pfaff, D.W. Estradiol regulation of estrogen receptor messenger ribonucleic acid in rat mediobasal hypothalamus: An in situ hybridization study. *J. Neuroendocrinol.* 2(5):605–611, 1990b

Lauber, A.H., Romano, G.J., Pfaff, D.W. Sex difference in estradiol regulation of progestin receptor mRNA in rat mediobasal hypothalamus as demonstrated by in situ hybridization. *Neuroendocrinology* 53:608–613, 1991b

LeDoux, J. *The emotional brain.* New York: Simon & Schuster, 1996

Lee, M., Donahoe, P., et al. Mullerian inhibiting substance in humans: Normal levels from infancy to adulthood. *J. Clin. Endocrinol. Metab.* 81(2):571–576, 1996

Lee, M., Donahoe, P., et al. Measurements of serum mullerian inhibiting substance in the evaluation of children with nonpalpable gonads. *N. Engl. J. Med.* 336(21):1480–1486, 1997

Legouis, R., Hardelin, J.P., Petit, C., et al. The candidate gene for the X-linked Kallmann syndrome encodes a protein related to adhesion molecules. *Cell* 67:423–435, 1991

Limouzin-Lamothe, M., Mairon, N., LeGal, J., LeGal, M., Quality of life after the menopause: Influence of hormonal replacement therapy. *Am. J. Obstet. Gynecol.* 170:618–624, 1994

Loeb, J. *Forced movements, tropisms and animal conduct.* Philadelphia: Lippincott, 1918

Lorenz, K. *Studies in animal and human behavior.* (R. Martin, Trans.). Cambridge, MA: Harvard University Press, 1970

Lu, R., Ko, H., Yao, B., et al. Lower level of estradiol in postpartum depression among Chinese women [abstract 504]. *Biol. Psychiatry* 39:648, 1996

Luine, V. Estradiol increases choline acetyltransferase activity in specific basal forebrain nuclei and projection areas of female rats. *Exp. Neurol.* 89:484–490, 1985

Luine, V.N. Steroid hormone influences on spatial memory. *Ann. N.Y. Acad. Sci.* 743:201–211, 1994

Luine, V. Estrogenic enhancements of and sex differences in memory in rats. *Soc. Behav. Neuroendocrinol* 44, 1997

Lund, S., Pompeiano, O. Monosynaptic excitation of alpha motoneurones from supraspinal structures in the cat. *Acta Physiol. Scand.* 54:270–286, 1968

Lustig, R.H., Pfaff, D.W., Mobbs, C.V. Two-dimensional gel autoradiographic analysis of the acute effects of estradiol on protein synthesis in the female rat ventromedial nucleus in vivo. *Endocrinology* 124:1863–1869, 1989

Lustig, R.H., Sudol, M., Pfaff, D.W., Federoff, H.J. Estrogenic regulation and sex dimorphism of growth-associated protein 43 kDa (GAP-43) messenger RNA in the rat. *Mol. Brain Res.* 11:125–132, 1991

Luttge, W. Intracerebral implantation of antiestrogen CN69, 725-27: Effects on female sexual behavior in rats. *Pharmacol. Biochem. Behav.* 4:685–688, 1976

Lydon, J.P., DeMayo, F.J., Funk, C.R., et al. Mice lacking progesterone receptor exhibit pleiotropic reproductive abnormalities. *Genes Dev.* 9:2266–2278, 1995

MacLean, P.D. Psychosomatic disease and the "visceral brain": Recent developments bearing on the Papez theory of emotion. *Psychosom. Med.* 11:338–353, 1949

MacLean, P.D. The triune brain: Emotion and scientific bias. In F.O. Schmidt (Ed.), *The neurosciences: Second study program*. New York: Rockefeller University Press, 1970:336–349

MacLean, P.D. *The triune brain in evolution: Role in paleocerebral functions*. New York: Plenum, 1990

Majewska, M.D., Harrison, N.L., Schwartz, R.D., Barker, J.L., Paul, S.M. Steroid hormone metabolites are barbiturate-like modulators of the GABA receptor. *Science* 232:1004–1007, 1986

Mani, S., Blaustein, J., O'Malley, B. Hormones and neurotransmitter interactions in behavior [abstract S43-3]. *Endo '97* 55, 1997

Maslow, A. The role of dominance in the social and sexual behavior of infrahuman primates: III. A theory of sexual behavior of infrahuman primates. *J. Genet. Psychology* 48:310–338, 1936

Maslow, A. *Motivation and personality*. New York: Harper, 1954

Matthews, T.J., Grigore, M., Tang, L., Kow, L-M., Doat, M., Pfaff, D.W. Sexual reinforcement in the female rat. *J. Experimental Analysis of Behavior* 68:399–410, 1997

McCarthy, M.M. Estrogen modulation of oxytocin and its relation to behavior. *Adv. Exp. Med. Biol.* 395:235–245, 1995

McCarthy, M.M. Chung, S.R., Ogawa, S., et al. Behavioral effects of oxytocin: Is there a unifying principle? In *Vasopressin* 208:195–212, 1991

McCarthy, M.M., Kleopoulus, S.P., Mobbs, C.V., Pfaff, D.W. Infusion of antisense oligodeoxynucleotides to the oxytocin receptor in the ventromeidal hypothalamus reduces estrogen-induced sexual receptivity and oxytocin receptor binding in the female rat. *Neuroendocrinology* 59:432–440, 1994

McCarthy, M.M. McDonald, C., Phillip, B., Goldman, D. An anxiolytic action of oxytocin is enhanced by estrogen in the mouse. *Physiol. Behav.* 60:1209–1215, 1996

McCarthy, M.M., Schlenker, E., Pfaff, D.W. Enduring consequences of neonatal treatment with antisense oligonucleotides to estrogen receptor mRNA on sexual differentiation of rat brain. *Endocrinology* 133:433–443, 1993

McCarthy, M.M., Schwartz-Giblin, S., Wang, S.M. Does estrogen facilitate social behavior by reducing anxiety? *Ann. N.Y. Acad. Sci.* 807:541–542, 1997

McCarthy, M.M., Chung, S.K., Ogawa, S., et al. Behavioral effects of oxytocin: Is there a unifying principle? *Vasopressin* 208:195–212, 1991b

McClintock, M.K. Menstrual synchrony and suppression. *Nature* 229:244–245, 1971

McEwen, B.S., Jones, K.J., Pfaff, D.W. Hormonal control of sexual behavior in the female rat: Molecular, cellular and neurochemical studies. *Biol. Reprod.* 36:37–45, 1987

McKenzie, J., Zakariza, M., Hyperthyroidism. In L. DeGroot (Ed.), *Endocrinology* (3rd ed.). Philadelphia: Saunders, 1995:676–711

McLaren, J., Prentice, A., Charnock-Jones, D.S., et al. Vascular endothelial growth factor is produced by peritoneal fluid macrophages in endometriosis and is regulated by ovarian steroids. *J. Clin. Invest.* 98:482–489, 1996

McMillan, P.J., Singer, C.A., Dorsa, D.M. The effects of ovariectomy and estrogen replacement on trkA and choline acetyltransferase mRNA expression in the basal forebrain of the adult female sprague-Dawley rat. *J. Neurosci.* 16:1860–1865, 1996

McQueen, J., Wilson, H., Fink, G. Estradiol-17β increases serotonin transporter (SERT) mRNA levels and the density of SERT-binding sites in female rat brain. *Mol. Brain Res.* 45: 13–23, 1997

Meisel, R.L., Pfaff, D.W. Specificity and neural sites of action of anisomycin in the reduction or facilitation of female sexual behavior in rats. *Horm. Behav.* 19:237–251, 1985

Meisel, R.L., Sachs, B.D. The physiology of male sexual behavior. In E. Knobil, J. Neill (eds.), *The physiology of reproduction* (2nd ed.). New York: Raven, 1994

Meyerson, B.J., Lindstrom, L. Sexual motivation in the estrogen treated ovariectomized rat. In V.H.T., James, L. Martini (Eds.), *Hormonal steroids (Proceedings of the Third International Congress on Hormonal Steroids, Hamburg, September 7–12, 1970)*. Amsterdam: Excerpta Medica, 1971:731–737

Michael, C., Kantor, H., Shore, H. Further psychometric evaluation of older women: The effect of estrogen administration. *J. Gerontol.* 25(4):337–341, 1970

Michael, R.P., Bonsall, R.W. Peri-ovulatory synchronisation of behaviour in male and female rhesus monkeys. *Nature (Lond.)* 265:463–465, 1977

Michael, R.P., Zumpe, D. Sexual initiating behaviour by female rhesus monkeys *(Macaca mulatta)* under laboratory conditions. *Behaviour* 36:168–186, 1970

Midgley, A.R., Jaffe, R.B. Regulation of human gonadotropins: IV. Correlation of serum concentrations of follicle stimulating and luteinizing hormones during the menstrual cycle. *J. Clin. Endocrinol. Metab.* 28:1699–1703, 1986

Miller, N.E. Liberalization of basic S-R concepts: Extensions to conflict behavior, motivation and social learning. In S. Koch (Ed.), *Psychology: A study of a science* (Study 1, Vol. 2). New York: McGraw-Hill, 1959:196–292

Miller, N.E. Behavioral and physiological techniques: Rationale and experimental designs for combining their use. In C.F. Code, W. Heidel (eds.), *Handbook of physiology, Sect. 6: Alimentary canal, Vol. 1.* Baltimore: Williams & Wilkins, 1967:51–61

Mobbs, C.V., Fink, G., Pfaff, D.W. HIP-70: A protein induced by estrogen in the brain and LH-RH in the pituitary. *Science* 247:1477–1479, 1990a

Mobbs, C.V., Fink, G., Pfaff, D.W. HIP-70: An isoform of phosphoinositol-specific phospholipase C-alpha. *Science* 249:566, 1990b

Mobbs, C.V., Harlan, R.E., Burrous, M.R., Pfaff, D.W. An estradiol-induced protein synthesized in the ventral medial hypothalamus and transported to the midbrain central gray. *J. Neurosci.* 8:113–118, 1988

Modianos, D., Pfaff, D.W. Brain stem and cerebellar lesions in female rats: II Lordosis reflex. *Brain Res.* 106:47–56, 1976

Modianos, D.T., Pfaff, D.W. Facilitation of the lordosis reflex in female rats by electrical stimulation of the lateral vestibular nucleus. *Brain Res.* 134:333–345, 1977

Moenter, S., Woodfill C., et al. Role of the thyroid gland in seasonal reproduction: Thyroidectomy blocks seasonal suppression of reproductive neuroendocrine activity in ewes. *Endocrinology* 128:1337–1344, 1991

Moenter, S., et al. *Endocrinology* 129:1175, 1991

Mohr, E., Bahnsen, U., Kiessling, C., Richter, D. Expression of the vasopressin and oxytocin genes in rats occurs in mutually exclusive sets of hyphothalamic neurons. *FEBS Lett*. 242:144–148, 1988

Mohr, E., Meyerhof, W., Richter, D. Vasopressin and oxytocin: Molecular biology and evolution of the peptide hormones and their receptors. *Vitam. Horm*. 51:235–266, 1995

Morgan, C.T. *Physiological psychology*. New York: McGraw-Hill, 1943

Morgan, M.A., Dellovade, T.L., Ogawa, S., Pfaff, D.W. Female mouse sexual behavior is regulated by thyroid hormones and estrogen [abstract]. *Soc. Neurosci. Abstr*. 1997

Morin, L., Dark, J. Hormones and biological rhythms. In L. Becker, S. Breedlove, D. Crews, (Eds.), *Behavioral endocrinology*. Cambridge, MA: MIT Press; 1994:473–504

Morin, L.P., Feder H.H. Hypothalamic progesterone implants and facilitation of lordosis behavior in estrogen-primed ovariectomized guinea pigs. *Brain Res*. 70:81–93, 1974

Morley, S., Christiane, S., Heierhorst, J., et al. Vasotocin genes of the teleost fish *Catostomus commersoni:* Gene structure, exon-intron boundary, and hormone precursor organization. *Biochemistry* 29:2506–2511, 1990

Morrell, J.I., Pfaff, D.W. A neuroendocrine approach to brain function: Localization of sex steroid concentrating cells in vertebrate brains. *Am Zool*. 18:447–460, 1978

Mortel, K.F., Meyer, J.S. Lack of postmenopausal estrogen replacement therapy and the risk of dementia. *J. Neuropsychiatr. Clin. Neurosci*. 7:334–337, 1995

Moss, R.L., Dudley, C.A. The challenge of studying the behavioral effects of neuropeptides. In L.L., Iversen., S.D., Iversen, S.H. Snyder (Eds.), *Handbook of psychopharmacology,* Vol. 18. New York: Plenum, 1984

Moss, R.L., Flynn, R.E., Shen, X.M., et al. Urine-derived compound evokes membrane responses in mouse vomeronasal receptor neurons. *J. Neurophysiol.* 77:2856–2862, 1997a

Moss, R.L., Gu, Q., Wong, M. Estrogen: Nontranscriptional signaling pathway. *Recent Prog. Horm. Res.* 52:1–37, 1997b

Moss, R.L., McCann, S.M. Induction of mating behavior in rats by luteinizing hormone releasing hormone. *Science* 181:177–179, 1973

Mountcastle, V.B. *Medical physiology,* Vol. 1 (13th ed.) St. Louis: Mosby, 1974

Moyer, K.E. *The psychobiology of aggression.* New York: Harper & Row, 1976

Nakano, K., Suga, S., Hishina, Y., et al. *Neurosci. Lett.* 225:17–20, 1997

Nauta, W.H.J., Karten, H.J. A general profile of the vertebrate brain, with sidelights on the ancestry of cerebral cortex. In F.O. Schmitt (Ed.), *The neurosciences: Second study program.* New York: Rockefeller University Press, 1970:7–276

Neumann, I., Russell, J.A., Landgraf, R. Oxytocin and vasopressin release within the supraoptic and paraventricular nuclei of pregnant, parturient and lactating rats: A microdialysis study. *Neuroscience* 53:65–75, 1993

Numan, M. Maternal behavior. In E. Knobil, J. Neill (Eds.), *The physiology of reproduction* (2nd ed.). New York: Raven, 1994:221–302

Nicot., A; Ogawa, S., Berman, Y.E., Carr, K.D., Pfaff, D.W. Effects of an acute intrahypothalamic injection of antisense oligonucleotides for preproenkephalin mRNA in female rats: Evidence for opioid involvement in lordosis. *Brain Res.,* in press, 1998

Ogawa, S., Gordan, J., Taylor, J., Lubahn, D., Korach, K., Pfaff, D. Reproductive functions illustrating direct and indirect effects of genes on behavior. *Horm. Behav.* 30:487–494, 1996a

Ogawa, S., Lubahn, D.B., Korach, K.S., Pfaff, D.W. Behavioral effects of estrogen receptor gene disruption in male mice. *Proc. Natl. Acad. Sci. U.S.A.* 94:1476–1481, 1997

Ogawa, S., Olazabal, U.E., Parhar, I.S., Pfaff, D.W. Effects of intrahypothalamic administration of antisense DNA for progesterone receptor mRNA on reproductive behavior and progesterone receptor immunoreactivity in female rat. *J. Neurosci.* 14:1766–1774, 1994

Ogawa, S., Taylor, J., Lubahn, D.B., Korach, K.S.,, Pfaff, D.W. Reversal of sex roles in genetic female mice by disruption of estrogen receptor gene. *Neuroendocrinology* 64:467–470, 1996b

Ohno, S., Christian, L., Attardi, B. Role of testosterone in normal female function. *Nature New Bio.* 243:119, 1973a

Ohno, S., Christian, L., Attardi, B., Kan, J. The modification of expression of the testicular feminization (Tfm) gene of the mouse by a "controlling element" gene. *Nature New Biol.* 245: 92, 1973b

Olias, G., Richter, D., Schmale, H. Heterologous expression of human vasopressin–neurophysin precursors in a pituitary cell line: Defective transport of a mutant protein from patients with familial diabetes insipidus. *DNA Cell Biol.* 15(11):929–935, 1996

Paganini-Hill, A. Estrogen replacement therapy and stroke. *Prog. Cardiovasc. Dis.* 38:223–242, 1995

Parhar, I.S., Iwata, M., Pfaff, D.W., Schwanzel-Fukuda, M. Embryonic development of gonadotropin-releasing hormone neurons in the sockeye salmon. *J. Comp. Neurol.* 362:256–270, 1995

Parhar, I.S., Iwata, M., Pfaff, D.W., Schwanzel-Fukuda, M. Gonadotropin-releasing hormone gene expression in teleosts. *Mol. Brain Res.* 41:216–227, 1996

Parsons, B., MacLusky, N.J., Krey, L., Pfaff, D. W., McEwen, B. S. The temporal relationship between estrogen-inducible progestin receptors in the female rat brain and the time course of estrogen activation or mating behavior. *Endocrinology* 107:774–779, 1980

Parsons, B., MacLusky, N.J., Krieger, M.S., McEwen, B. S., Pfaff, D. W. The effects of long-term estrogen exposure on the induction of sexual behavior and measurements of brain estrogen and progestin receptors in the female rat. *Horm. Behav.* 301–313, 1979

Parsons, B., McEwen, B.S., Pfaff, D.W. A discontinuous schedule of estradiol treatment is sufficient to activate progesterone-facilitated feminine sexual behavior and to increase cytosol receptors for progestins in the hypothalamus of the rat. *Endocrinology* 110:613–619, 1982a

Parsons, B., Rainbow, T.C., Pfaff, D.W., McEwen, B.S. Oestradiol, sexual receptivity and cytosol progestin receptors in rat hypothalamus. *Nature* 292:58–59, 1981

Parsons, B., Pfaff, D.W. Progesterone receptors in CNS correlated with reproductive behavior. *Cur. Top. Neuroendocrinol.* 5:103–140; 1985

Parsons, B., Rainbow, T., Pfaff, D.W., McEwen, B.S. Hypothalamic protein synthesis essential for the activation of the lordosis reflex in the female rat. *Endocrinology* 110:620–624, 1982b

Pau, K.-Y., et al., *Endocrinology.* 133:1650, 1993

Pauly, P. *Controlling life: The engineering ideal in biology.* New York: Oxford University Press, 1987

Pedersen, C., Caldwell, J., Jirikowski, G., Insel, T. Oxytocin in maternal, sexual, and social behaviors. *Ann. N.Y. Acad. Sci.* 652:1992

Penrose, R. *The emperor's new mind: Concerning computers, minds and the laws of physics.* New York: Oxford University Press, 1989

Peterson, B.W. Distribution of neural responses to tilting within vestibular nuclei of the cat. *J. Neurophysiol.* 33:750–767, 1970

Pfaff, D.W. Cerebral implantation and autoradiography studies of sex hormones. In J. Money (Ed.), *Sex research: New developments.* New York: Holt, Rinehart & Winston, 1965:219–234

Pfaff, D.W. Autoradiographic localization of radioactivity in rat brain after injection of tritiated sex hormones. *Science* 161:1355–1356,1968a

Pfaff, D.W. Uptake of estradiol-17B-H3 in the female rat brain. An autoradiography study. *Endocrinology* 82:1149–1155, 1968b

Pfaff, D.W. Mating behavior of hypophysectomized rats. *J. Comp. Physiol. Psychol.* 72:45–50, 1970a

Pfaff, D.W. Nature of sex hormone effects on rat sex behavior: Specificity of effects and individual patterns of response. *J. Comp. Physiol. Psychol.* 73:349–358,1970b

Pfaff, D.W. Luteinizing hormone releasing factor (LRF) potentiates lordosis behavior in hypophysectomized ovariectomized female rats. *Science* 182:1148–1149, 1973

Pfaff, D.W. *Estrogens and brain function: Neural analysis of a hormone-controlled mammalian reproductive behavior.* New York: Springer-Verlag, 1980

Pfaff, D.W. Neurobiological mechanisms of sexual motivation. In D.W. Pfaff, (Ed.), *The physiological mechanisms of motivation.* New York: Springer-Verlag, 1982a:287–317

Pfaff, D.W. (Ed.). *The physiological mechanisms of motivation.* New York:Spring-Verlag, 1982b

Pfaff, D.W. Multiplicative responses to hormones by hypothalamic neurons. In S. Yoshida, L. Share (Eds.), *Recent progress in posterior pituitary hormones.* Amsterdam: Elsevier Science, 1988:257–267

Pfaff, D.W. Patterns of steroid hormone effects on electrical and molecular events in hypothalamic neurons. *Mol. Neurobiol.* 3:135–154, 1989

Pfaff, D.W. Hormones, genes, and behavior. *Proc. Natl. Acad. Sci. USA* 94:14213–14216, 1997

Pfaff, D.W., Cohen, R.S. Estrogen acting on hypothalamic neurons may have trophic effect on those neurons and the cells on which they synapse. In P.C.K. Leung et al. (Eds.), *Endocrinology and physiology of reproduction.* New York: Plenum 1987:1–11

Pfaff, D.W. Conrad, L.C.A. Hypothalamic neuroanatomy: Steroid hormone binding and patterns of axonal projections. *Int. Rev. Cytol.* 54:245–265, 1978

Pfaff, D.W., Lewis, C. Film analyses of lordosis in female rats. *Horm. Behav.* 5:317–335, 1974

Pfaff, D.W., Modianos, D. Neural mechanisms of female reproductive behavior. In R. Goy, N. Adler D.W. Pfaff (Eds.) *Neurobiology of Reproduction* New York: Plenum, 1980

Pfaff, D.W., Peyser, E.R. Molecular studies of hormone-dependent brain mechanisms in relation to the drive concepts of psychoanalysis. In U. Halbreich (Ed.), *American Psychiatric Association Press Series on Hormones and Behavior* (in press)

Pfaff, D.W., Pfaffmann, C. Olfactory and hormonal influences on the basal forebrain of the male rat. *Brain Res.* 15:137–156, 1969

Pfaff, D.W., Gerlach, J., McEwen, B.S., et al. Autoradiographic localization of hormone-concentrating cells in the brain of the female rhesus monkey. *J. Comp. Neurol.* 170:279–294,1976

Pfaff, D.W., Keiner, M. Atlas of estradiol-concentrating cells in the central nervous system of the female rat. *J. Comp. Neurol.* 151:121–158, 1973

Pfaff, D.W., Kow, L.-M., Zhu, Y.-S., et al. Hypothalamic cellular and molecular mechanisms helping to satisfy axiomatic requirements for reproduction. *J. Neuroendocrinol.* 8:325–336, 1996.

Pfaff, D.W., Lewis, C., Diakow, C., Keiner, M. Neurophysiological analysis of mating behavior responses as hormone-sensitive reflexes. *Prog. Physiol. Psychol.* 5:253–297, 1972

Pfaff, D.W., Montgomery, M., Lewis, C. Somatosensory determinants of lordosis in female rats: Behavioral definition of the estrogen effect. *J. Comp. Physiol. Psychol.* 91:134–145, 1977

Pfaff, D.W., Schwartz-Giblin, S., McCarthy, M.M., Kow, L.-M. Cellular and molecular mechanisms of female reproductive behaviors. In E. Knobil, J. Neill (Eds.), *The physiology of reproduction* (2nd ed.). New York: Raven, 1994:107–220

Pfaff, D.W., Zigmond, R.E. Neonatal androgen effects on sexual and nonsexual behavior of adult rats tested under various hormone regimes. *Neuroendocrinology* 7:129–145, 1971

Pfaus, J.G., Jakob, A., Kleopoulos, S.P., Gibbs, R.B., Pfaff, D.W. Sexual stimulation induces *Fos* immunoreactivity within GnRH neurons of the female rat preoptic area: Interaction with steroid hormones. *Neuroendocrinology* 60:283–290, 1994

Pfaus, J.G., Kleopoulos, S.P., Mobbs, C.V., Gibbs, R.B., Pfaff, D.W. Sexual stimulation activates c-*fos* within estrogen-concentrating regions of the female rat forebrain. *Brain Res.* 624: 253–267, 1993

Pfaus, J.G., Pfaff, D.W. Mu, delta, and kappa opioid receptor agonists selectively modulate sexual behaviors in the female rat: Differential dependence on progesterone. *Horm. Behav.* 26: 457–473, 1992

Phillips, S.M., Sherwin, B.B. Effects of estrogen on memory function in surgically menopausal women. *Psychoneuroendocrinology* 17:485–495, 1992a

Phillips, S.M., Sherwin, B.B. Variations in memory function and sex steroid hormones across the menstrual cycle. *Psychoneuroendocrinology* 17:497–506, 1992b

Picazo, O., Fernandez-Guasti, A. Anti-anxiety effects of progesterone and some of its reduced metabolites: An evaluation using the burying behavior test. *Brain Res.* 680:135–141, 1995

Pleim, E., Brown, T., MacLusky, N., et al. Dilute estradiol implants and progestin receptor induction in the ventromedial nucleus of the hypothalamus: Correlation with receptive behavior in female rats. *Endocrinology* 124:1807–1812, 1989

Priest, C.A., Borsook, D., Pfaff, D.W. Estrogen and stress interact to regulate the hypothalamic expression of a human proenkephalin promoter-β-galactosidase fusion gene in a site-specific and sex-specific manner. *J. Neuroendocrinol.* 9:317–326, 1996

Quiñones-Jenab, V., Jenab, S., Ogawa, S., Adan, R.A.M., Burbach, P.H., Pfaff, D.W. Effects of estrogen on oxytocin receptor messenger ribonucleic acid expression in the uterus, pituitary and forebrain of the female rat. *Neuroendocrinology* 65:9–17, 1997

Quiñones-Jenab, V., Jenab, S., Ogawa, S., Funabashi, T., Weesner, G.D., Pfaff, D.W. Estrogen regulation of gonadotropin-releasing hormone receptor messenger RNA in female rat pituitary tissue. *Mol. Brain Res.* 38:243–250, 1996

Quiñones-Jenab, V., Jenab, S., Ogawa, S., Inturrisi, C., Pfaff, D.W. Estrogen regulation of mu-opioid receptor messenger RNA in the forebrain of female rats. *Mol. Brain Res.* (in press)

Quiñones-Jenab, V., Ogawa, S., Jenab, S., Pfaff, D.W. Estrogen regulation of preproenkephalin messenger RNA in the forebrain of female mice. *J. Chem. Neuroanat.* 12:29–36, 1996

Quiñones-Jenab, V., Zhang, C., Jenab, S., Brown, H.E., Pfaff, D.W. Anesthesia during hormone administration abolishes the estrogen induction of preproenkephalin mRNA in ventromedial hypothalamus of female rats. *Mol. Brain Res.* 35:297–303, 1996

Rance, N., Uswandi, S. Gonadotropin-releasing hormone gene expression is increased in the medial basal hypothalamus of postmenopausal women. *J. Clin. Endocrinol. Metab.* 81(10):1–7, 1996

Rance, N., Young, W. Hypertrophy and increased gene expression of neurons containing neurokinin-B and substance-P messenger ribonucleic acids in the hypothalami of postmenopausal women. *Endocrinology* 128:2239–2247, 1991

Rance, N., McMullen, N., Smialek, J., et al. Postmenopausal hypertrophy of neurons expressing the estrogen receptor gene in the human hypothalamus. *J. Clin. Endocrinol. Metab.* 71(1):79–85, 1990

Rance, N., Young, W., McMullen, N. Topography of neurons expressing luteinizing hormone-releasing hormone gene transcripts in the human hypothalamus and basal forebrain. *J. Comp. Neurol.* 339:573–586, 1994

Rhodes, C.H., Morrell, J.L., Pfaff, D.W. Distribution of estrogen-concentrating, neurophysin containing magnocellular neurons in the rat hypothalamus as demonstrated by a technique combining thyroid autoradiography and immunohistology in the same tissue. *Neuroendocrinology* 33:18–23, 1981

Rhodes, C.H., Morrell, J.I., Pfaff, D.W. Estrogen-neurophysin-containing hypothalamic magnocellular neurons in the vasopressin-deficient (Brattleboro) rat: A study combining steroid autoradiography and immunocytochemistry. *J. Neurosci.* 2:1718–1724, 1982

Ricciardi, K.H., Blaustein, J.D. Projections from ventrolateral hypothalamic neurons containing progestin receptor–and substance p–immunoreactivity to specific forebrain and midbrain areas in female guinea pigs. *J. Neuroendocrinol.* 6:135–144, 1994

Richard, S., Zingg, H.H. The human oxytocin gene promoter is regulated by estrogens. *J. Biol. Chem.* 265:1–6, 1990

Richards, R.G., DiAugustine, R., Petrusz, P., et al. Estradiol stimulates tyrosine phosphorylation of the insulin-like growth factor-1 receptor and insulin receptor substrate-1 in the uterus. *Proc. Natl. Acad. Sci. U.S.A.* 93:12002–12007, 1996

Richards, S., Beck, K., Luine, V. Object recognition task performance in rats: Sex difference and estrogen treatment effects. *Soc. Behav. Neuroendocrinol.* 136, 1997

Risold, P., Swanson, L. Structural evidence for functional domains in the rat hippocampus. *Science* 272:1484–1486, 1996

Robbins, T.W., Everitt, B.J. Arousal systems and attention. In M. Gazzaniga et al. (Eds.), *Handbook of cognitive neuroscience.* Cambridge; MA:MIT Press, 1996:703–720

Roberts, J.L., Dutlow, C.M., Jakubowski, M., et al. Estradiol stimulates preoptic area–anterior hypothalamic proGnRH-GAP gene expression in ovariectomized rats. *Mol. Brain. Res.* 6:127–134, 1989

Rodriguez-Sierra, J., Howard, J., Pollard, G., Hendricks, S. Effect of ovarian hormones on conflict behavior. *Psychoneuroendocrinology* 9:293–300, 1984

Romano, G.J., Harlan, R.E., Shivers, B.D., Howells, R.D., Pfaff, D.W. Estrogen increases proenkephalin messenger ribonucleic acid levels in the ventromedial hypothalamus of the rat. *Mol. Endocrinol.* 2:1320–1328, 1988

Romano, G.J., Krust, A., Pfaff, D.W. Expression and estrogen regulation of progesterone receptor mRNA in neurons of the mediobasal hypothalamus: An *in situ* hybridization study. *Mol. Endocrinol.* 3:1295–1300, 1989.

Romano, G.J., Mobbs, C.V., Howells, R.D., Pfaff, D.W. Estrogen regulation of proenkephalin gene expression in the ventromedial hypothalamus of the rat: Temporal qualities and synergism with progesterone. *Mol. Brain Res.* 5:51–58, 1989b

Romano, G.J., Mobbs, C.V., Lauber, A., Howells, R.D., Pfaff, D.W. Differential regulation of proenkephalin gene expression by estrogen in the ventromedial hypothalamus of male and female rats: Implications for the molecular basis of a sexually differentiated behavior. *Brain Res.* 536:63–68, 1990

Rosie, R., Thomson, E., Fink, G. Oestrogen positive feedback stimulates the synthesis of LHRH mRNA in neurones of the rostral diencephalon of the rat. *J. Neuroendocrinol.* 8:185–191, 1990

Ross, J. Basic/clinical symposium: Gonadal steroids and the brain. *Endo '97*, The Endocrine Society. p. 54, 1997

Ross, G.T., Cargille, C.M., Lipsett, M.B., et al. Pituitary and gonadal hormones in women during spontaneous and induced ovulatory cycles. *Recent Prog. Horm. Res.* 26:1–48, 1970

Rothfeld, J., Hejtmancik, J.F., Conn, P.M., Pfaff, D.W. In situ hybridization for LHRH mRNA following estrogen treatment. *Mol. Brain Res.* 6:121–125, 1989

Rowe, D.W., Erskine, M.S. c-*Fos* proto-oncogene activity induced by mating in the preoptic area, hypothalamus, and amygdala in the female rat: Role of afferent input via the pelvic nerve. *Brain Res.* 621:25–34, 1993

Roy, E., Wade, G. Binding of ^{3}H-estradiol by brain cell nuclein and female sexual behavior: Inhibition by antiestrogens. *Brain Res.* 126:73–87, 1977

Roy, E., Lynn, D.M., Clark, A.S. Inhibition of sexual receptivity by anesthesia during estrogen priming. *Brain Res.* 337:163–166, 1985

Rubin, B., Barfield, R. Induction of estrous behavior in ovariectomized rats by sequential replacement of estrogen and progesterone to the ventromedial hypothalamus. *Neuroendocrinology* 37:218–224, 1983a

Rubin, B., Barfield, R. Progesterone in the ventromedial hypothalamus facilitates estrous behavior in ovariectomized estrogen-primed rats. *Endocrinology* 113:797–804, 1983b

Rubin, B., Barfield, R. Progesterone in the ventromedial hypothalamus of ovariectomized, estrogen-primed rats inhibits subsequent facilitation of estrous behavior by systemic progesterone. *Brain Res.* 294:1–8, 1984

Rubinow, D., Schmidt, P. Reproductive hormones and mood in women [abstract 386]. *Biol. Psychiatry* 39:613, 1996

Russell, J.A., Douglas, A.J., Bull, P., et al. Pregnancy and opioid interactions with the anterior peri–third ventricular input to magnocellular oxytocin neurones. *Prog. Brain Res.* 91:41–53, 1992

Russell, J.A., Leng, G., Bicknell, R.J. Opioid tolerance and dependence in the magnocellular oxytocin system: A physiological mechanism? *Exp. Physiol.* 80:307–340, 1995a

Russell, J.A., Douglas, A.J., Bull, P.M., et al. Changing interactions of opioids with oxytocin neurones in pregnancy. In T. Saito, K. Kurokawa, S. Yoshida (Eds.), *Neurohypophysis: Recent progress of vasopressin and oxytocin research. Proceedings of the First Joint World Congress of Neurohypophysis and Vasopressin.* Amsterdam: Elsevier 1995b:275–288,

Sakai, R., Ma, L., Zhang, D., et al. Intracerebral administration of mineralocorticoid receptor antisense oligonucleotides attenuate adrenal steroid-induced salt appetite in rats. *Neuroendocrinology* 64:425–429, 1996

Sakai, R., Nicolaidis, S., Epstein, A. Salt appetite is suppressed by interference with angiotensin II and aldosterone. *Am. J. Physiol.* 251:R762–R768, 1986

Sakamoto, Y., Suga, S., Sakuma, Y. *J. Neurophysiol.* 70:1469–1475, 1993

Sakuma, Y. *J. Physiol. (Lond.)* 349:273–286, 1984

Sakuma, Y. *Horm. Behav.* 28:438–444, 1994

Sakuma, Y., Akaishi, T. *J. Neurophysiol.* 57:1148–1159, 1987

Sakuma, Y., Pfaff, D.W. Facilitation of female reproductive behavior from mesencephalic central gray in the rat. *Am. J. Physiol.* 237:R278–R284, 1979a

Sakuma, Y., Pfaff, D.W. Mesencephalic mechanisms for integration of female reproductive behavior in the rat. *Am. J. Physiol.* 237:R285–R290, 1979b

Sakuma, Y., Pfaff, D.W. *J. Neurophysiol.* 44:1002–1011, 1980a

Sakuma, Y., Pfaff, D.W. Convergent effects of lordosis-relevant somatosensory and hypothalamic influences on central gray cells in the rat mesencephalon. *Exp. Neurol.* 70:269–281, 1980b

Sakuma, Y., Pfaff, D.W. Excitability of female rat central gray cells with medullary projections: Changes produced by hypothalamic stimulation and estrogen treatment. *J. Neurophysiol.* 44:1012–1023, 1980c

Sakuma, Y., Pfaff, D.W. LLH-RH in the mesencephalic central gray can potentiate lordosis reflex of female rats. *Nature* 283:566–567 1980d

Sakuma, Y., Pfaff, D.W. *Brain Res.* 225:184–188, 1981

Sakuma, Y., Pfaff, D.W. *Exp. Brain Res.* 46:292–300, 1982

Sakuma, Y., Pfaff, D.W. Modulation of the lordosis reflex of female rats by LHRH, its antiserum and analogs in the mesencephalic central gray. *Neuroendocrinology* 36:218–224, 1983

Sakuma, Y., Tada, T. *J. Physiol. (Lond.)* 349:287–297, 1984

Sarkar, D., Chiappa, S., Fink, G. *Nature* 264:461, 1976

Sato, Y., et al., *Exp. Brain Res.* 112:197–202, 1996

Sato, H., Okawa, T., Uchino, Y., Wilson, V.J. Excitatory connections between neurons of the central cervical nucleus and vestibular neurons in the cat. *Exp. Brain Res.* 115(3):381–386, 1997

Selye, H. *Stress without distress.* Philadelphia: Lippincott, 1974

Schechter, D., Bachmamm, G., Vaitukaitis, J., et al. Perimenstrual symptoms: Time course of symptom intensity in relation to endocrinologically defined segments of the menstrual cycle. *Psychosom. Med.* 51:173–194, 1989

Schechter, D., Strasser, T., Endicott, J., et al. Role of ovarian steroids in modulating mood in premenstrual syndrome [abstract 499]. *Biol. Psychiatry* 39:646, 1996

Schmale, H., Richter, D. Single base depletion in the vasopressin gene is the cause of diabetes insipidus in Brattleboro rats. *Nature* 308:705–709, 1984

Schmidt, P., Berman, K., Leibenluft, E., et al. The neuregulatory consequences of hypogonadism [abstract S43-2]. *Endo '97* 55,: The Endocrine Society, 1997

Schmidt, P., Nieman, L., Danaceau, M., et al. Differential behavioral effects of gonadal steroids in women with and in those without premenstrual syndrome. *N. Engl. J. Med.* 338: 209–216, 1998

Schumacher, M., Baulieu, E. Neurosteroids: Synthesis and functions in the central and peripheral nervous systems. In Ciba Foundation Symposium 191, *Non-reproductive actions of sex steroids.* 90–112 Chichester, NY: Wiley, 1995:

Schumacher, M., Coirini, H., Pfaff, D.W., McEwen, B.S. Behavioral effects of progesterone associated with rapid modulation of oxytocin receptors. *Science* 250:691–694, 1990

Schumacher, M., Coirini, H., Pfaff, D.W., McEwen, B.S. Light-dark differences in behavioral sensitivity to oxytocin. *Behav. Neurosci.* 105(3):487–492, 1991

Schumacher, M., Coirini, H., Johnson, A.E., Flanagan, L.M., Frankfurt, M., Pfaff, D.W. McEwen, B.S. The oxytocin receptor: A target for steroid hormones. In F. Legros et al. (Eds.), *Regulatory peptides,* Vol. 45. New York: Elsevier, 1993:115–119

Schumacher, M.H., Coirini, D.W., Pfaff, D.W., McEwen, B.S. Localized actions of progesterone in hypothalamus involve oxytocin. *Proc. Natl. Acad. Sci. U.S.A.* 86:6798–6801, 1989

Schwanzel-Fukuda, M., Abraham, S., Crossing, K.L., Edelman, G.M., Pfaff, D.W. Immunocytochemical demonstration of neural cell adhesion molecule (NCAM) along the migration route of luteinizing hormone-releasing hormone (LHRH) neurons in mice. *J. Comp. Neurol.* 321:1–18, 1992a

Schwanzel-Fukuda, M., Abraham, S., Reinhard, G.R., Crossin, K.L., Edelman, G.M., Pfaff, D.W. Antibody to neural cell adhesion molecule (NCAM) can disrupt the migration of luteinizing hormone–releasing hormone (LHRH) neurons into the mouse brain. *J. Comp. Neurol.* 342:174–185, 1994

Schwanzel-Fukuda, M., Bick, D., Pfaff, D.W. Luteinizing hormone–releasing hormone (LHRH)–expressing cells do not migrate normally in an inherited hypogonadal (Kallmann) syndrome. *Mol. Brain Res.* 6:311–326, 1989

Schwanzel-Fukuda, M., Crossin, K.L., Pfaff, D.W., Boulox, P.M.G., Hardelin, J.P.,, Petit, C. Migration of LHRH neurons in early human embryos: Association with neural cell adhesion molecules. *J. Comp. Neurol.* 366:547–557, 1996

Schwanzel-Fukuda, M., Jorgenson, K., Bergen H., Weesner, G., Pfaff D.W. Biology of normal LHRH neurons during and after their migration from olfactory placode. *Endocr. Rev.* 13(4):623–633, 1992b

Schwanzel-Fukuda, M., Pfaff, D.W. Origin of luteinizing hormone–releasing hormone neurons. *Nature* 338:161–164, 1989

Schwanzel-Fukuda, M., Pfaff, D.W. Combination of tritiated thymidine autoradiography and neuropeptide immunocytochemistry to determine birth dates and migration routes of luteinizing hormone–releasing hormone neurons. In P. Michael Conn (Ed.) *Methods in Neurosciences,* Vol. 3. New York: Academic Press, 1990:90–106

Scott, R.E.M., Wu-Peng, S., Kaplitt, M.G., Pfaff, D.W. In vivo promoter analysis of the rat progesterone receptor using an HSV viral vector [abstract 704.16]. *Soc. Neurosci. Abstr.* 1790, 1996

Scott, R.E.M., Wu-Peng, S., Yen, P.M., Chin, W.W.,, Pfaff, D.W Comparison of a progesterone receptor estrogen response element with the consensus ERE in their ability to respond to thyroid hormone receptors. *Mol. Endocrinol.* 11:1581–1592, 1997

Sherrington, C. *The integrative action of the nervous system.* New Haven: Yale University Press, 1906

Sherwin, B.B. Estrogenic effects on memory in women. *Ann. N.Y. Acad. Sci.* 743:213–231, 1994

Sherwin, B.B. Hormones, mood and cognitive functioning in postmenopausal women. *Obstet. Gynecol.* 87:20S–26S, 1996

Sherwin, B.B., Tulando, T. "Add-back" estrogen reverses cognitive deficits induced by a gonadotropin-releasing hormone agonist in women with leiomyomata uteri. *J. Clin. Endocrinol. Metab.* 81:2545–2549, 1996

Shifren, J.L., Tseng, F., Zaloudek, C.J., et al. Ovarian steroid regulation of vascular endothelial growth factor in the human endometrium: Implications for angiogenesis during the menstrual cycle and in the pathogenesis of endometriosis. *J. Clin. Endocrinol. Metab.* 81:3112–3118, 1996

Shivers, B., Harlan, R., Morrell, J., Pfaff, D.W. Absence of oestradiol concentration in cell nuclei of LHRH-immunoreactive neurones. *Nature* 304:345–347, 1983

Shizuta, Y., Kawamoto, T., Mitsuuchi, Y., et al. Inborn errors of aldosterone biosynthesis in humans. *Steroids* 60(1):15–21, 1995

Sichel, D., Cohen, L., Robertson, L., et al. Prophylactic estrogen in recurrent postpartum affective disorder. *Biol. Psychiatry* 38:814–818, 1995

Silverman, A., Izhar, L., Witkin, J. The gonadotropin releasing hormone (GnRH) neuronal systems: Immunocytochemistry and in situ hybridization. In E. Knobil, J. Neill (Eds.), *The physiology of reproduction* (2nd ed.), New York: Raven, 1994:1683–1710

Simerly, R.B., Carr, A.M., Zee, M.C., Lorang, D. Ovarian steroid regulation of estrogen and progesterone receptor messenger ribonucleic acid in the anteroventral periventricular nucleus of the rat. *J. Neuroendocrinol.* 8:45–56, 1996

Simerly, R.B., Chang, C., Muramatsu, M., Swanson, L.W. Distribution of androgen and estrogen mRNA-containing cells in the rat brain: An in situ hybridization study. *J. Comp. Neurol.* 294:76–95, 1990

Singer, C.A., Pang, P.A., Dobie, D.J., Dorsa, D.M. Estrogen increases GAP-43 (neuromodulin) mRNA in the preoptic area of aged rats. *Neurobiol. Aging* 17:661–663, 1996a

Singer, C.A., Rogers, K.L., Strickland, T.M., Dorsa, D.M. Estrogen protects primary cortical neurons from glutamate toxicity. *Neurosci. Lett.* 212:13–16, 1996b

Smith, M.S., Freeman, M.E., Neill, J.D. The control of progestin secretion during the estrous cycle and early pseudopregnancy in the rat: Prolactin, gonadotropin and steroid levels associated with rescue of the corpus luteum of pseudopregnancy. *Endocrinology* 96:219–226, 1975

Smith, M., Zuoxin, W., Luskin, M., Insel, T. Estrus induction associated with neurogenesis in the brain of female prairie voles. *Soc. Behav. Neurosci.* 110:174, 1997

Smith, S.S. Estrous hormones enhance coupled, rhythmic olivary discharge in correlation with facilitated limb stepping. *Neuroscience* 82(1), 1997:271–283

Sodersten, P., Eneroth, P., Mode, A. Gustaffson J.-A. Mechanisms of androgen-activated sexual behaviour in rats. In R. Gilles, J. Balthazart (Eds.), *Neurobiology*. Berlin: Springer-Verlag. 1985:48–59

Stahl, S. Reproductive hormones as adjuncts to psychotropic medications [abstract 388]. *Biol. Psychiatry*. 39:613, 1996

Stellar, E. Brain mechanisms in hunger and other hedonic experiences. *Proc. Am. Philos. Soc.* 118:276–282, 1974

Stern, K., McClintock, M. Regulation of ovulation by human pheromones. *Nature* 392: 177–179, 1998

Stopa, E., Koh, E., Svendsen, C., et al. Computer-assisted mapping of immunoreactive mammalian gonadotropin-releasing hormone in adult human basal forebrain and amygdala. *Endocrinology* 128:3199–3207, 1991

Strong, O.S., Elwyn, A. In R.C. Truex, M.B. Carpenter (Eds.), Human anatomy (5th ed.). Baltimore: Williams & Wilkins; 1964:8

Suga, S., Sakuma, Y. *Brain Res. Bull.* 33:205–210, 1994

Sukhov, R., Walker, W., Rance. N., et al. Vasopressin and oxytocin gene expression in the human hypothalamus. *J. Comp. Neurol.* 337:295–306, 1993

Sukhov, R., Walker, W., Rance. N., et al. Opioid precursor gene expression in the human hypothalamus. *J. Comp. Neurol.* 353:604–622, 1995

Sulloway, F.J. *Freud, biologist of the mind*. Cambridge, MA: Harvard University Press, 1979

Suzuki, J.-I., Cohen, B. Head, eye, body and limb movements from semicircular canal nerves. *Exp. Neurol.* 10:393–405, 1964

Takeo, T., Sakuma, Y. *Neurosci. Res.* 22:73–80, 1995

Tang, M., Jacobs, D., Stern, Y., et al. Effect of estrogen during menopause on risk and age at onset of Alzheimer's disease. *Lancet* 348:429–432, 1996

Tannenbaum, P., Wallen, K. Sexually initiated affiliation facilitates rhesus monkey integration. *Ann. N.Y. Acad. Sci.* 807:578–582, 1997

Teixeira, J., Donahoe, P., et al. Developmental expression of a candidate müllerian inhibiting substance type II receptor. *Endocrinology* 137(1):160–165, 1996

ten Bruggencate, G., Lundberg, A. Facilitory interaction in transmission to motoneurones from vestibulospinal fibres and contralateral primary afferents. *Exp. Brain Res.* 19:248–270, 1974

Tetel, M.J., Calentano, C., Blaustein, J.D. Intraneuronal convergence of tactile and hormonal stimuli associated with female reproduction in rats. *J. Neuroendocrinol.* 6:211–215, 1994

Thibaut, F., Cordier, B., Kuhn, J.M. Modulation medicamenteuse de la libido et de l'activite sexuelle. Effet comportemental d'un analogue de la GnRH chez l'homme. *Ann. Endocrinol.* 55:229–233, 1994

Thrun, L., Dahl, G., et al. A critical period for thyroid hormone action on seasonal changes in reproductive neuroendocrine function in the ewe. *Endocrinology* 138:3402–3409, 1997

Tinbergen, N. *The Study of instinct.* London: Oxford University Press, 1951 *Understanding and preventing violence,* Vols. 1–4. Washington: National Academy Press, 1994

Toran-Allerand, C.D., Hashimoto, K., Greenough, W.T., Saltarelli, M. Sex steroids and the development of the newborn mouse hypothalamus and preoptic area in vitro: III. Effects of estrogen on dendritic differentiation. *Brain Res.* 283:97–110, 1983

Utiger, R. Hypothroidism. In L. DeGroot (Ed.), *Endocrinology (3rd ed.)* Philadelphia: Saunders, 1995: 752–768

Valentino, R., Foote, S., Page, M. The locus coeruleus as a site for integrating corticotropin-releasing factor and noradrenergic mediation of stress responses. *Ann. N.Y. Acad. Sci.* 697: 173–187, 1993

Vanderhorst, V., Holstege, G. Estrogen induces axonal outgrowth in the nucleus retro-ambiguus-lumbosacral motoneuronal pathway in the adult female cat. *J. Neurosci.* 17:1122–1136, 1997

van Oortmerssen, G.A., Bakker, T.C.M. Artificial selection for short and long attack latencies in wild *Mus musculus domesticus. Behav. Genet.* 11:115–126, 1991

Vathy, I., Etgen, A., Barfield, R. Actions of progestins on estrous behavior in female rats. *Physiol. Behav.* 40:591–595, 1987

Vathy, I., Etgen, A., Barfield, R. Actions of RU 38486 on progesterone facilitation and sequential inhibition of rat estrous behavior: Correlation with neural progestin receptor levels. *Horm. Behav.* 23:43–56, 1989

Wade, J., Arnold, A. Functional testicular tissue does not masculinize development of the zebra finch song system. *Proc. Natl. Acad. Sci. U.S.A.* 93:5264–5268, 1996

Walker, W., Feder, H. Antiestrogen effects on estrogen accumulation in brain cell nuclei: Neurochemical correlates of estrogen action on female sexual behavior in guinea pigs. *Brain Res.* 134:467–478, 1977a

Walker, W., Feder, H. Inhibitory and facilitatory effects of various antiestrogens on the induction of female sexual behavior by estradiol benzoate in guinea pigs. *Brain Res.* 134:455–465, 1977b

Wallen, K., Nature needs nurture: The interaction of hormonal and social influences on the development of behavioral sex differences in rhesus monkeys. *Horm. Behav.* 30(4):364–378, 1996

Wallen, K., Tannebaum, P. Hormonal modulation of sexual behavior and affiliation in rhesus monkeys. *Ann. N.Y. Acad. Sci.* 807:185–202, 1997

Warembourg, M., Poulain, P., Presence of estrogen receptor immunoreactivity in the oxytocin-containing magnocellular neurons projecting to the neurohypophysis in the guinea pig. *Neuroscience* 40:41–53, 1991

———

Warner, L.H. A study of sex behavior in the white rat by means of the obstruction method. *Comp. Psychol. Monogr.* 4:1–66, 1927

Watson, J., Crick, F.H.C. Genetical implications of the structure of deoxyribonucleic acid. *Nature* 177:964, 1953

Webster, J., Moenter, S., et al. Role of the thyroid gland in seasonal reproduction. II. Thyroxine allows a season-specific suppression of gonadotropin secretion in sheep. *Endocrinology* 129:176–183, 1991a

Webster, J., Moenter, S., et al. Role of the thyroid gland in seasonal reproduction. III. Thyroidectomy blocks seasonal suppression of gonadotropin-releasing hormone secretion in sheep. *Endocrinology* 129:1635–1643, 1991

Weiland, S., Lan, N., Mirasedeghi, S., Gee, K. Anxiolytic activity of the progesterone metabolite 5α-pregnan-3α-ol-20-one. *Brain Res.* 565:263–268, 1991

Wetsel, W.C. Immortalized hypothalamic luteinizing hormone-releasing hormone (LHRH) neurons: A new tool for dissecting the molecular and cellular basis of LHRH physiology. *Cell. Mol. Neurobiol.* 15:43–78, 1995

Wide, L., Nillius, S.J., Gemzell, C., Roos, P. Radioimmunosorbent assay of follicle stimulating hormone and luteinising hormone in serum and urine from men and women. *Acta Endocrinol.* (Copenh.) 74:1–60, 1973

Wilson, E.O. *On human nature.* Cambridge, MA: Harvard University Press, 1978

Wilson, J.D. Metabolism of testicular androgens. In R.O. Greep, E.B.Astwood (Eds.), *Handbook of physiology, Vol. 5.* Washington, DC: American Physiological Society; 1975: 491–508

Wilson, J.D., George, F.W., Renfree, M.B. The endocrine role in mammalian sexual differentiation. *Recent Prog. Horm. Res.* 50:349–64, 1995

Wilson, J.D., Griffin, J.E., Russell, D.W. Steroid 5α-reductase 2 deficiency. *Endocr. Rev.* 14:577–593, 1993

Wilson, V.J. Physiology of the vestibular nuclei. In R.F. Naunton (Ed.) *The vestibular system.* New York Academic 1975:109–128

Wilson, V.J. The labyrinth, the brain and posture. *Am. Sci.* 63:325–332, 1967

Wilson, V.J., Yoshida, M. Comparison of effects of stimulation of Deiter's nucleus and medial longitudinal fasciculus on neck, forelimb, and hindlimb motoneurons. *J. Neurophysiol.* 32:743–758, 1969

Wilson, V.J., Yoshida, M., Schor, R.H. Supraspinal monosynaptic excitation and inhibition of thoracic back motoneurons. *Exp. Brain Res.* 11:282–295, 1970

Windle, R.J., Shanks, N., Lightman, S.L., Ingram, C.D. Central oxytocin administration reduces stress-induced corticosterone release and anxiety behavior in rats. *Endocrinology* 138:2829–2834, 1997

Witt, D.M. Regulatory mechanisms of oxytocin-mediated sociosexual behavior. *Ann. N.Y. Acad. Sci.* 807:287–301, 1997

Witt, D.M., Insel, T.R. A selective oxytocin antagonist attenuates gonadal steroid facilitation of female sexual behavior. *Endocrinology* 128:3269–3276, 1991

Witt, D.M., Insel, T.R. Central oxytocin antagonism decreases female reproductive behavior. *Ann. N.Y. Acad. Sci.* 652:445–447, 1992

Wood, R., Newman, S. Androgen and estrogen receptors coexist within individual neurons in the brain of the Syrian hamster. *Neuroendocrinology* 62:487–497, 1995

Woolley, C.S. Hormone-induced structural plasticity in the adult hippocampus. *Soc. Behav. Neuroendocrinol.* 46, 1997

Woolley, C.S., Gould, E., Frankfurt, M., McEwen, B.S. Naturally occurring fluctuation in dendritic spine density on adult hippocampal pyramidal neurons. *J. Neurosci.* 10:4035–4039, 1990

Woolley, C.S., McEwen, B.S. Estradiol mediates fluctuation in hippocampal synapse density during the estrous cycle in the adult rat. *J. Neurosci.* 12:2549–2554, 1992

Woolley, C.S., McEwen, B.S. Estradiol regulates hippocampal dendritic spine density via an N-methyl-D-aspartate receptor-dependent mechanism. *J. Neurosci.* 14:7680–7687, 1994

Wotjak, C.T., Masaharu, K., Liebsch, G., et al., Release of vasopressin within the rat paraventricular nucleus in response to emotional stress: A novel mechanism of regulating adrenocorticotropic hormone secretion. *J. Neurosci.* 16:7725–7732, 1996

Yamaguchi, K., Akaishi, T., Negoro, H. Effects of estrogen treatment on plasma oxytocin and vasopressin in ovariectomised rats. *Endocr.J.* 26:197–205, 1979

Yamashita, H., Okuya, S., Inenaga, K., et al. Oxytocin predominately excites putative oxytocin neurons in the rat supraoptic nucleus in vitro. *Brain Res.* 416:364–368, 1987

Yin, J., Kaplitt, M.G., Kwong, A.D., Pfaff, D.W. In vivo promoter analysis for detecting an estrogen effect on preproenkephalin (PPE) transcription in hypothalamic neurons [abstract 471] *Endocr. Soc. Abstr.* 318, 1994

Yin, J., Kaplitt, M.J., Pfaff, D.W. In vivo promoter analysis in the adult central nervous system using viral vectors. In M.J. Kaplitt, A.D. Loewy (Eds.), *Viral vectors*: Gene therapy and neuroscience applications. New York: Academic, 1995: 157–171

Yoshida, M., Suga, S., Sakuma, Y. *Exp. Brain Res.* 101:1–7, 1994

Young, P.T. *Motivation of behavior.* New York: Wiley, 1936

Zadina, J.E., Kastin, A.J., Fabre, L.A., Coy, D.H. Facilitation of sexual receptivity in the rat by an ovulation-inhibiting analog of LHRH. *Pharmacol. Biochem. Behav.* 15:961–964, 1981

Zhang, Y., Proenca, R., Maffei, M. Barone, M., Leopold, L., Friedman, J.M. Positional closing of the mouse obese gene and its human homologue. *Nature* 372:425–432, 1994

Zhu, Y.-S., Pfaff, D.W. DNA binding of hypothalamic nuclear proteins on estrogen response element and preproenkephalin promoter: Modification by estrogen. *Neuroendocrinology* 62: 454–466, 1995.

Zhu, Y.-S., Dellovade, T.L.,, Pfaff, D.W. Gender-specific induction of pituitary RNA by estrogen and its modification by thyroid hormone. *J. Neuroendocrinol.*9:395–403, 1997

Zhu, Y.-S., Ling, Q., Cai, L.Q., Imperato-McGinley, J.,, Pfaff, D.W.Regulation of pre-proenkephalin (PPE) gene expression by estrogen and its interaction with thyroid hormone [Abstract] *Soc. Neurosci. Abstr.* 1997b

Zhu, Y.S., Yen, P., Chin, W.W., Pfaff, D.W. Estrogen and thyroid hormone interaction on regulation of gene expression. *Proc. Natl. Acad. Sci. U.S.A.* 93:12587–12592, 1996

Zigmond, R.E., Detrick, R.A., Pfaff, D.W. An autoradiographic study of the localization of androgen concentrating cells in the chaffinch. *Brain Res.* 182:369–381, 1980

Zigmond, R.E., Nottebohm, F., Pfaff, D.W. Androgen-concentrating cells in the midbrain of a songbird. *Science* 179:1005–1007, 1973

Zumpe, D., Michael, R.P. Ovarian hormones and female sexual invitations in captive rhesus monkeys (*Macaca mulatta*). *Anim. Behav.* 18:293–301, 1970

Index

Note: Figures are indicated by an italic *f* after page numbers, tables by an italic *t*.